RHYTHMS of LIFE

Why We Do the Things We Do When We Do

PETER WEST

GREEN MAGIC

Rhythms of Life © 2021 by Peter West. All rights reserved. No part of this book may be used or reproduced in any form without written permission of the author, except in the case of quotations in articles and reviews.

Green Magic
53 Brooks Road
Street
Somerset
BA16 0PP
England

www.greenmagicpublishing.com

Designed & typeset by K.DESIGN
Winscombe, Somerset

ISBN 9781838132446

GREEN MAGIC

CONTENTS

1	INTRODUCTION	5
2	THE THEORY AND DEVELOPMENT OF BIORHYTHMS	11
3	THE PHYSICAL CYCLE	27
4	THE EMOTIONAL CYCLE	43
5	THE INTELLECTUAL CYCLE	55
6	CALCULATIONS	67
7	THE DAILY BIORHYTHMS	85
8	COMPATIBILITY	95
9	PRACTICAL CYCLES	109
10	THE RHYTHMS OF LIFE	123
11	THE RHYTHMS OF NATURE	135
12	THE INTUITIONAL CYCLE AND OTHER RHYTHMS	147
13	THE SPORTING WORLD	161
14	CELEBRITY LIST	169

CHAPTER 1

INTRODUCTION

We humans have been created with all manner of recurring continuous emotional, intellectual and physical rhythms that just never stop. In essence, we are in fact a vast collection of never-ending cyclic changes within the tiniest cells of our physical bodies, our organic makeup and in our behavioural attitudes.

Because we have grown so used to them, the vast majority of us are probably quite unaware of them so that when or what things do happen along these lines, we tend to accept them and may not recognise such matters as cyclic events. For example, look at the way we breathe and accept the way our hearts, kidney and liver functions keep us going. Most of us are active during the day but rest at night. It is also how we cope with the ever changing seasons of spring, summer, autumn and winter that we all more or less take within our daily stride, as a matter of course. Equally, probably just as many of us are totally unaware.

Some of us accept these events as a matter of course. A few of us may fight them, but many of us are quite unaware that there are a lot more of these rhythms that we do not even know about yet. In amongst all these series of continuous changes, there are three now quite clearly defined cycles that affect out behaviour patterns although, in themselves, they have no cause and effect as such. They are continuous physiological changes that we all experience and to which we all respond in some way or another. They govern the way we think and reason matters through, the way we respond emotionally and the ups and downs of our physical responses.

There are now known to be several other cycles that can and do affect the way we behave, and we will mention them later in the chapter on other cycles. Clever researchers have also found that we respond to certain cycles when two of these main rhythms are viewed together. In effect, they have found extra cycles that affect our overall behaviour patterns, but that is all looked at later.

These three main cycles are recognised collectively as biorhythms and are individually called the physical cycle, with a duration of 23 days; the sensitivity (or emotional) cycle, with a periodicity of 28 days; and the intellectual cycle lasting 33 days.

These three principal rhythms appear to control or hold sway over our performance in three distinct areas of behaviour. But it must be stressed that none of them have any direct cause and effect in themselves. In each case, they tend to fall subject to the prevailing conditions of the environment of the moment.

Research has shown that there is a correlation between the state of these individual cycles and certain factors in our behaviour. As time has progressed, we are now much more aware of how the stage or phase of each of these rhythms allows an individual the opportunity to correct or adjust his or her conduct accordingly. The success rate following such action has been phenomenal.

So, biorhythm cycles are most certainly one answer to the behaviour patterns we experience in our 'on' or 'off' days and the proper application and awareness of these phases help to provide a much more positive approach to life.

Biorhythms do not indicate that, at a specific time, this may happen or that an accident will occur. They don't indicate

INTRODUCTION

that you will win a sweepstake or that you will change your occupation. They do, however, indicate the state of your present physical ability, the condition of your emotional sensitivity or the standard of your intellect on a particular day.

It is what you do with this knowledge that is the real key to understanding and using biorhythms. How you apply what you have learned concerning such capabilities or limitations in each of the three cycles at any given time is entirely a matter of your personal choice.

THE THREE PRINCIPAL RHYTHMS

Each of the three rhythms start on the day you were born and remain constant until you die. They are known respectively as the Physical Cycle which appears to regulate our physical abilities and limitations, the Emotional Rhythm which seems to have an effect on the way we respond emotionally, and the Intellectual Cycle which holds sway over the way we reason things through.

Because of their regularity, it is possible to calculate their individual phases or stages quite easily for any particular day: past, present or even for future events. All that is needed is your date of birth.

Now this will bring a criticism that there is link or a comparison with astrology but this has yet to be proved. While both disciplines, that is astrology or biorhythms, deal with the individual and that those people may be advised on the right path or attitude to take at certain times, astrology advises in more different terms. Biorhythms, on the other hand, can only provide you with your (probable) state of mind in respect of your abilities and limitations at the time.

However, for a few folk, biorhythms often appear the more accurate of the two but you must not take this as a sleight against astrology. In this case, the two concepts are quite different and there is no hidden or magical interpretation involved. Biorhythms are, quite simply, an exercise in calculating a physiological function and relating the result to the behaviour pattern of the individual concerned.

COMPATIBILITY

Shortly after the theory of biorhythms became public knowledge, it was obviously only a question of time before they became subjected to a fairly diverse field of all kinds of experiments. By far and away the most popular of these was the study of compatibility.

Because your personal biogram, that is the chart we create to illustrate the stages of your individual cycles, reveals your potential behaviour patterns, it follows that what they 'do' for you, they must 'do' for others. Thus, the logical step is to compare these charts and by studying them it becomes quite easy to see how we ought to get along with others. It is not infallible by any means, but most of the time we can see why we cannot get along with him, but we can get along with her.

To exist in this rather complex modern world, we must get along with others to the best of our ability, but this is not as easy as it sounds. We may find ourselves behaving strangely toward a man or woman we have just met for the first time. Somehow, something does not quite 'click' into place and the relationship does not get off to a very good start. At other times, we find that we get along swimmingly, as if we had always been friends. A notable rapport is created. Sometimes, people we have known for a long time seem to rub us up the wrong way and there may not be any easy answer as to why.

When we start to compare the biograms of the individuals concerned, it soon becomes evident to see why we do get along with him but not her. This is not an infallible system by any means, but most of the time we can see why this may

INTRODUCTION

be so. This special study does not have all the answers, but they can, and often do, provide an illuminating insight into a relationship. The almost limitless possibilities here show that human behavioural patterns and potential compatibility are capable of being compared and that the results obtained are as equally exciting.

Elsewhere, the clever use of biorhythms has been successfully employed in safety in all forms of transport and the wide variety of sporting arenas. The mass of incredible results found have had managers, trainers and coaches singing the praises of biorhythms to the high heavens. Where steps have been taken to do so, accident rates have fallen quite dramatically in each these fields of endeavour – truly a remarkable success story.

In the following pages you will find all the information you will need to calculate and show you that not only can and do the three principal biorhythms help you live a better life, but also the many other cycles that have been discovered add their influences as well.

Planning with and using these cycles will not only be personally helpful to you, but will also allow you to understand precisely what is making the other person behave the way they are on any particular day.

Just think how useful that can be to help make you live a more productive life.

CHAPTER 2

THE THEORY AND DEVELOPMENT OF BIORHYTHMS

Life of all kind responds in some way to rhythmic behavioural patterns because of the inner natural cycles that have an influence from either an external source or from inside the body. By far and away the most recognised rhythm or cycle known to man must be day and night and how we tend to respond this natural and regular phenomenon.

Generally speaking, most life forms, including man, more or less obey it without question. The majority of people and animals sleep and or just rest during the hours of darkness because they are mostly diurnal creatures. Those who live by night are what we call nocturnal creatures and for them this procedure is reversed.

For some time we have been aware of the many other cycles and rhythms that affect us. The most natural of these are the seasons, which follow on from day and night. We have to start somewhere, so why not with new life? So, come the spring, we see fresh life appear in the animal and plant kingdoms and as we move through to summer we note that life grows and flourishes in abundance. As we proceed through the autumn, some life starts to prepare for either hibernation or death. This is usually when life forms of just about all shapes and sizes tend to stay fairly dormant awaiting the return of spring, when the life giving Sun returns and whole cycle starts all over again.

However, not everything responds so readily to this rather fundamental periodicity. Some animal life flourishes quite well during the winter and may even take on the appearance of a totally different animal. Perhaps the most notable of these would be the stoat and ermine – one and the same creature in reality, but one that has differing responses to nature and its rhythms according to the season.

As the seasons change, so does the outward appearance of this animal. This is no haphazard change for there is a clearly defined traceable pattern marking the distinctive changes in this animal's life cycle. It is when these changes are checked against statistical evidence recorded over long periods of time and then transcribed into graphs and updated that what changes do occur are much more easily traceable. The complete life cycle of the ermine and stoat emerges in such predictable ways that the overall picture can be seen and absorbed by anyone.

Cyclic behavioural patterns regarding human life should not be confused with the natural rhythms of man. Behavioural patterns evolve through the way in which we develop and live. When these are recorded, the results have shown some extraordinary statistics that may be illustrated in the following series of crime information that were collated during the period between the two World Wars of the last century.

In America, statistics were compiled from the law office files of some 2000 plus towns and cities over a period of five years. It was discovered that the information yielded curious links between seasonal changes and crime patterns. The data appeared to be so accurate that one of the chiefs of the F.B.I. was reported as suggesting that meteorologists obviously had the ability to predict rapes as well as storms but to a limited degree of course.

These patterns varied very little from one year to the next. Nevertheless, it was found that there were more murders that seemed to occur during July and August than at any other time, especially at weekends. More than 60% of these killings took place between 18:00 hours and 06:00 hours. Burglary, however, was a different proposition. Between 18:00 hours and 02:00 hours on Saturday nights in December, January and February seemed to be the most favoured times for this activity. May produced very little serious crime, other than for an increase in attacks by dogs. Suicides chose June more than at any other time and where there were any; recordings of such admissions were reported to hospitals. Curiously, there were also more marriages in this month as well. February and November saw an upsurge in more cars being stolen than at any other time.

Perhaps it is worth noting at this stage, that around 3000 years ago the Greek physician, Hippocrates, observed that human beings seemed to experience good days and bad. Unfortunately, we are unable to find out if there were any studies made to support the claim. However, we do know that this assumption was recorded as being irrespective of whether people were ill or not. It is quite probable this theory had been studied and discussed earlier but it appears that it was regarded as less important than it now is to know, register and study these good or bad spells.

HERMANN SWOBODA

Shortly before the end of the 19th century, Hermann Swoboda, a professor at the University of Vienna, became aware of a certain traceable type of regularity in some of man's attitudes. He watched, waited and observed. At last, among other equally important discoveries, he realised that there was a definite rhythmical periodicity which seemingly affected man and his behavioural patterns.

Professor Swoboda continued his research in order to establish whether this fluctuating phenomenon could be predetermined by calculation in some way. Further, he then set out to prove this and finally arrived at the existence of a 23-day cycle which seemed to affect man's physical, behavioural reactions.

Research refined the professor's findings in respect of this cycle. At about this same time, Swoboda also discovered a 28-day cycle of emotional reaction and behaviour. This second rhythm was not as easily discernible as the first one because it seemed to coincide with the menstrual cycle in women.

However, because a similar periodicity was observable in men, Swoboda was keen to prove the existence of such a clearly defined pattern and, of course, irrespective of the natural rhythm of a woman. His painstaking research was rewarded by convincing evidence of these cycles of life.

Although he was more of a psychologist than a scientist per se, Swoboda was quite gifted with a natural analytical and systematic mind and, once he became reasonably sure of his findings, he published his first book, PERIODICITY IN MAN'S LIFE, followed by STUDIES IN THE BASIS OF PSYCHOLOGY. He also devised a very basic measuring system and an instruction booklet, THE CRITICAL DAYS OF MAN, to supplement it: the study of biorhythms had been born.

WILHELM FLIESS

In a sense, biorhythms had two parents although, quite curiously, neither was aware of the other at this particular birth. Through yet another one of life's curious coincidences and while Swoboda was conducting his research from his psychological point of view, another doctor was amassing and assessing similar information from the standpoint of a practising physician.

THE THEORY AND DEVELOPMENT OF BIORHYTHMS

Wilhelm Fliess, a Berlin nose and throat specialist, had observed the 23- and 28-day cyclic behavioural patterns for himself. He was one of the first to realise, or at least to publicly pronounce upon a possible correlation between biorhythms and behavioural patterns.

His beliefs were founded upon the simple theory that each of us inherits both male and female characteristics and that everyone probably had some trace of bisexuality in their make-up. Fliess was quite sure of his findings and published his findings in his book, THE COURSE OF LIFE. Sadly, this exciting new work went largely unrecognised at the time.

It was dismissed as being a tad too complex and mathematical for the layman (or anyone else for that matter) to understand what he was proposing but this did not prevent him from continuing his researches. He realised the importance of his discoveries and discussed them frequently with another giant of his time, Sigmund Freud, who became so convinced of the validity of Fliess's work that he began to use his colleague's theories in his own practice. During the development of Freud's now famous pscho-analytical ideologies, the Fliess theories were frequently referred to and employed.

However, these were early days yet and like most new ideas and theories, the struggle for acceptance proved to be a long and difficult task. Even today, many people find it hard to cope with the newest theories published in some fields of endeavour. It was far from easy during those early days of discovery to persuade others to accept what a researcher in any field was trying to prove.

Strange too for these Victorian times because so many people of the era were almost always ready to jump on the bandwagon for the possibility of the money involved and or to further their own personal fame. In the past hundred years or so, man's scientific knowledge has advanced significantly.

Computer technology is one good example. Around 50 or so years ago, a machine capable of the same functions as the modern mobile phone or tablet which most of us now carry around, would have occupied a space four or five metres square. With the silicon chip revolution now well established, the mobile phone and the portable tablet have fast developed into mini-computers in their own right.

With the machines – some barely wrist watch size in the early days of 2017, one might be forgiven for wondering in what direction these fields of technology were leading to.

In the early part of the 20th century, new theories were almost always treated initially with a mixture of prejudice, scorn and suspicion before even a minimal acceptance was achieved. Fliess and Swoboda had much to contend with but, despite traces of a grudging acceptance here or an outright repudiation there, they continued to build on their respective theories. They both produced masses of documentation and statistics.

Swoboda's massive work, THE YEAR OF SEVEN, contained mathematical analyses of the 23- and 28-day rhythmical repetitions displayed by subjects through several generations. It was vast in concept and represents the foundations on which modern biorhythmics (bio-chronobiology) are based. Today, with almost all computers, whether the mobile, lap-top or of the desk variety usually carry a program to take care of the tedious calculations. The only question mark against all this development is the wide variety of interpretation presented.

ALFRED TELTSCHER

Wilhelm Fliess died in the late 1920's, about the time when the third biorhythmic cycle was recognised. This time, the theorist was an engineer and a student of mathematics, Alfred Teltscher. There is very little hard evidence stemming authoritatively from Teltscher himself but it does appear that he developed and finally established the pattern for the 33-day cycle. This was after many years studying the many variations presented by his students' intellectual capacity.

He was able to show convincing and definite predetermined periods when people possessed poor perception and performance in their intellectual pursuits. Equally, he also noted that there were times when people more easily grasped new concepts, performed well and generally exhibited their intellectual acuity.

Further to this, two doctors, a Rexford Hersey and a Michael John Bennett at the Pennsylvania University, conducted similar research and, quite independently, arrived at similar conclusions regarding the intellectual cycle. So, once again, there was this curious coincidence occurring at the birth and discovery of this biorhythm.

CALCULATION

However, as with the recognition of the two previous rhythms, nothing really happened. There was no widespread use of biorhythms and the study was more or less driven into the side lines where it remained neglected for a long while, only occasionally being referred to in the ensuing years. One of the many reasons for this unfortunate neglect has been attributed to the apparently complicated calculations necessary for verifying the stages or phases of the cycles. None of the original pioneers seemed to have been able to simplify the methods that were employed in any way that would have proved acceptable to the layman and professional alike. Yet, in practice, the calculations are very simple.

Basically, all we have to do is count up the number of days that the individual has been alive. By counting the birthdate as one, all that is needed is the total number of days from the date of birth up to and including the day in question. The total is divided by the number of days in the required cycle; that is, 23 days for the physical, 28 days for the sensitivity and 33 days for the intellectual. These days, the intuitional cycle of 38 days should also now be included. In each case, the remainder figure (if there is one) that results from these divisions shows the stage of the individual rhythm. Where there is no remainder, the day in question is the start of the new cycle. The quick and easy way to pursue this figure work is fully detailed in the chapter on calculations.

Yet there appears to have been a stumbling-block or mystery attached to this area of biorhythmic study. Admittedly, some clumsy attempts at a satisfactory formula were made: slide rules were produced by various individuals; sets of complicated tables were published by those interested in the theory of biorhythms or as a result of the mathematical challenge presented by the problem.

Whatever the reason, interest declined although, with the exception of a few dedicated individuals. the whole concept seemed to just lurk in the pending file until, in 1939, interest was again aroused as the result of a new publication.

HANS SCHWING

In 1939, a Swiss doctor of the Federal Institute of Technology published a short study of accidents and accidental deaths that clearly showed a pattern, as predicted by these three biorhythms. In essence, the publication showed that after a study of some 700 accident cases and 300 cases of accidental death there was a strong correlation in respect of biorhythms.

Over a period of some 21,252 days ($23 \times 28 \times 33$) he isolated the critical days for the 23-day physical cycle, the 28-day emotional cycle, and the 33-day intellectual cycle. He illustrated that 322 accidents occurred during single critical days (in other words, one of the person's biorhythms were crossing the neutral line into positive or negative territory). 72 occurred on double critical days and five took place on triple critical days.

In total, he showed that of 401 accidents, 60% of all the incidents happened on critical days. The maximum total of critical days possible during a 21,252-day period is 4,427 days. That is 20% of the 21,252 days. Thus, 60% of accidents occurred at 20% of the times that coincided with the critical points.

In 1954, a report by a doctor Rheinhold Bochow of the Humboldt University in Berlin showed that out of 497 accidents, 97.8% of these took place on a critical day of one of the three body rhythms; 26.6% happened on single critical days; 46.5% on double critical days and 24.7% occurred on triple critical days.

A low-key public interest in biorhythmic studies was once again displayed, occasionally illustrated by an odd publication or two, but there seems to be very little reason for the sudden explosion of popularity that the subject has enjoyed in the last 40 to 50 years or so. Now, there is hardly a country in the world that does not have at least one biorhythm society or association. In the last few years, public interest in England has developed enormously. However we, in the UK, have not quite reached the stage in America where one can obtain a weekly forecast from a slot machine for a few cents.

There were a couple or so respected and well-conducted researchers and publications with some occasional publicity in newspapers to help the cause. One magazine used to offer a 'Readers' Biorhythm Service' for a very reasonable fee but the response was eventually considered to be too little to warrant further expense and time and it was passed on to private hands.

So, here we are, 150 years or so on from the original concept. Now we have an established, respected study and practice, which, provided it is properly employed, can and does lead to very significant improvements in the way we live. The next logical question is: do these rhythms affect us, how are they determined and what exactly are they?

It is of paramount importance to realise that the three cycles of biorhythms, irrespective of their phase, do not have a cause and effect in themselves. Fundamentally, they are continuous, physiological changes and awareness of them can help you to plan your way of life much more effectively. Because of the phasing of these cycles, you will either tend to perform well or give less than average attendance to matters of the moment subject to prevailing conditions.

Each rhythm begins on the day you are born and continues its individual course throughout life, only ceasing at death. Everyone has them and is 'subject' to their influence but just a tiny percentage of people do not 'conform' to the established patterns all the time.

The first half of each cycle is the plus, ascending, developing and progressive period. Confident and aggressive, full of vim and vigour, mental perception at a peak, you will perform well until you reach the zenith of your powers half way through this first phase. Your capabilities tend to remain at this high level but gradually tail off until the rhythm reverts to the second half of its cycle.

This second phase is the rejuvenation period, as though it were a recuperative period after an operation. This half of the cycle sinks to a nadir, again at the midpoint, then begins to steadily progress towards the positive phase once more until the cycle has been completed. The pattern is repeated, continuously, throughout life.

CRITICAL DAYS

The days on which the cycles begin or change from one phase to the other, are known as 'critical' days. Publicity of these days or, perhaps more accurately, the label 'critical' which has been applied to them, seems to have served to popularise biorhythms more than any other aspect. It has been proved, statistically, that accidents are more likely to occur on these critical days than at any other point in the cycles.

We have shown elsewhere that the probability of an incident or an accident occurring on these days is very high, whether through lowered physical vitality, irrational emotional behaviour or inferior mental perception causing the subject to be more accident prone.

There are several significant points in each of the cycles and they are detailed in the chapters which deal with the individual rhythms. The designation 'critical' is somewhat of a misnomer. However, nothing really critical does occur save for the actual changes in the cycles. In most aspects of life, the transition from one phase to another may be termed a turning point, a psychological moment, favourable or providential; or, perhaps, disturbing, unlucky, inauspicious or unsuitable, depending on individual circumstances.

Understanding that these various meanings can be applied to the critical days in your biorhythms will enable you to utilise them to your advantage. A change of job may, for example, be favourable in the greater analysis, but it is also disturbing. When a child leaves junior school to attend senior school, it is a turning point in his or her academic career, but it may also prove unsuitable because of the environmental changes involved. A new manager may be appointed to take charge of your department, shop or factory at a psychological moment favourable or unfavourable to you.

A change in a regular facet of life may, therefore, have an effect that can be determined in some cases, but only guessed at in others. Abrupt changes are a different matter altogether, however. Let us assume that you return home each day in exactly the same manner whatever the circumstances, irrespective of weather conditions, season or whatever.

For example, one day your regular train is cancelled, something that has never occurred before, or a party of tourists may be occupying the carriage you normally use. Your immediate reaction will be self-defensive, quite natural in the circumstances but it may manifest in different ways according to the individual personality. Despite the way in which you react in such a situation, you will be temporarily off-balance.

Perhaps you have arranged to meet someone at a specific time and place, with no doubts that the details of the meeting are correct. You arrive a few minutes early but, after twenty minutes or so, you realise that the other party is not going to arrive. Your most probable reaction will be one of temporary emotional disturbance and perhaps intellectual annoyance at suddenly being faced with an unexpected alternative to rectify such an unfamiliar situation.

Maybe you have planned and worked very hard to produce a sales programme which, you believe, cannot fail because of the untold hours you have spent verifying all the details. However, your boss rejects your scheme out of hand, either with qualifying his or her decision or perhaps not even bothering to give you a reason at all. Your inner reaction will leave you temporarily off-balance.

Such everyday situations, and your reactions to them, are what critical days are concerned with. You are temporarily off-balance during these transitional periods which can last for between 24 and 48 hours: a long time to be off-balance – even to a minor degree.

Suppose that one of the examples quoted above occurred while your biorhythms were in one of their transitional periods, you were experiencing a critical day, a double critical day or, even worse, a triple critical day. In such an event, your normal mode of behaviour could be swept aside in a moment of emotional irrationality, intellectual blindness or physical rage – you would be disturbed.

There is one point in everybody's life when all three biorhythms reach the same phase and stage as the day of birth, and they each restart their respective cycles all over again in exactly the same patterns. This 'grand triple critical day' occurs every 21,252 days or 58.2 years (58 years and 66 or 67 days if an extra leap year is involved) from the date of birth.

In this period, 924 physical cycles, 759 sensitivity cycles and 644 intellectual cycles have occurred. The figure 21,252 is arrived at by multiplying the number of days in each cycle together: 23 × 28 × 33. Up until this point, each rhythm has had a succession of critical days, sometimes coinciding with the other rhythms passing from either from the positive to the negative or from the negative to the positive phase. This will have resulted in double or triple critical days, but without all three cycles reaching the identical point as on the day of birth.

There are at least six critical days each month in everyone's biorhythms. Occasionally, there are eight. If you allow for the basic six occurring in an average month of thirty days, this means you are in a critical phase of your biorhythms for 20 per cent of your life, every month.

During the grand biorhythmic span of 58.2 years, there are many occasions when a double critical day occurs in the emotional and physical rhythms and it is this particular combination which is statistically proven to be the most accident-prone period. A single critical day portends a problem all its own of course because you are likely to be temporarily off-balance on this day. However, the emotional/

physical double critical days should be treated with more caution. Awareness of the inherent problems of these days may help prevent distress or accidents.

Simply checking back to a date when something went wrong has more than a 60 per cent probability of showing you were in a critical phase on that day. More to the point, you may even recall saying at the time that had you been 'aware' of certain information, the incident may not have happened.

In the physical rhythm, the critical days are 1 and 12; in the emotional cycle, on days 1 and 15; and intellectually, on days 1 and 17. There is a strong possibility that the date you are investigating may fall on or either side of these critical days, but there could be a simple explanation for this.

Your time of birth may have been very early in the morning and, while many doubt the validity of the actual birth time being important in this respect, others regard it as vital. There is some evidence that, where the timing of a critical day seems to be out by 24 hours, the time of birth is the best factor to consider. Similarly, a very late time of birth could have an effect in the opposite direction.

Alternatively, of course, it may be possible that you have the wrong date for your birthday. It may seem strange in this modern world with all its advanced technology to make such a suggestion, but it can and does happen all too frequently for the analyst to ignore the possibility. At this point, it would be wise to remember that biorhythms are not the 'be-all and end-all' of accuracy. Errors can occur but, statistically, the chances are strong that they will not.

Now, let us consider how biorhythms can be utilised for planning ahead. If you have important dates or events coming up in the future and wish to know your capabilities, it is a simple matter to check the particular phasing of your rhythms for such a time and plan accordingly.

Should the relevant cycle appear unfavourable, allow for the possibility of error in your behavioural patterns or, if you can change the proposed date to a more favourable time: then do so. A simple adjustment is all that is needed. Once again, there may be the inevitable comparison with astrology but you should disregard this, for there is no correlation yet proven. Despite all the advances which have been made in psychological analyses of behavioural patterns, an element of 'chance' could still possibly enter the equation.

STATISTICAL EVIDENCE

If the results of these accident statistics were to be used as the basis for future analyses by, say, a small transport company then surely the possibility of accidents could be reduced? Drivers could be taken off the road on their most accident-prone days or be asked to take on a different task. They could even be taught the fundamentals of biorhythmic theory in order to become more aware of the potential hazards of particular days in their cycles.

A company with good employer/employee relationships could even work out a rest-day rota system so that no real hardship would be involved either in earnings or in the loss, however temporary of personal prestige. This is exactly the sort of scheme which has been implemented by some companies all over the world. All kinds of business concerns, not only those directly concerned with transportation, have utilised biorhythmic studies in respect of their staff; the success rates achieved speak for themselves.

Accident figures are down, the insurance companies are more than happy, management are delighted and personnel involved feel the better for it. All this has led to increased productivity, which is an additional bonus.

Biorhythms can also be used effectively to check compatibility with others. We all want to get along as well as possible with other people, but this is not always easy to accomplish. However, we might as well make the best of what we can so, if there is a way of improving relationships, then the obvious step is to use whatever mode of improvement is available.

Your personal biograms reveal your potential behaviour patterns and, therefore, it must follow that if they do so for you, they do so for others also. The logical next step, then, is to compare them.

In the field of biorhythmic compatibility studies an astonishing success rate has been recorded once the basic principles have been understood and simple rules observed. The use of biorhythms does not stop here, however. They can be used to control diets, helping to stop smoking, improving sexual harmony, working to achieve better sporting success or making academic studies so much easier. You name the activity and we can apply the theory of biorhythms to it to help you improve all manner of tasks.

All you need to do is to have your personal cycles charted and from there the list of what to do and when to do it becomes endless.

CHAPTER 3

THE PHYSICAL CYCLE

The physical cycle concerns itself with the way we carry out all of our activities requiring the best possible method of performance and capability that we can summon at the time. Quite obviously, therefore, there is an enormous range of possibilities which, even when taken into consideration with the other two rhythms, must rate very high. This is because whatever you want to do at any time, the sheer physical ability to perform such tasks really ought to be as favourable as possible for a positive result to be attained.

There are times when this ability is required that the effects of the rhythm are barely noticeable while at others, it will be painfully obvious that all is not well. Therefore, during the course of our daily routine, it doesn't matter what day we select but it does help when we know what our physical ability for that time might be.

THE POSITIVE PHASE

Here we will show what might be considered a normal day when the physical cycle is in its positive stage. You hear your alarm begin to clatter and shatter the silence of the early hours and your arm reaches out to stop the dreadful racket. After you manage to find the stop button, you pause for a moment and you will either leap out ready for the day ahead or you will stagger out of your bed probably, as many thousands of us normally do.

When in the positive phase of this rhythm, you will awake feeling good. The men will start to shave reasonably easily irrespective of what they use, for their skin feels smooth warm and elastic. Those of them who use a blade find that it glides over the face with little trouble and they respond to an aftershave toner that sets them up for the day. The ladies will find their make-up much easier to apply which will make them feel that little extra special.

When this rhythm is in its positive stage you are more likely to have some kind of breakfast. You will enjoy your normal repast without too much trouble. Your journey to work will be rather easy. The short walk to the station will be accomplished with little effect and you will pass other folk who, on other days, have passed you. You won't mind having to stand on the train and, once at the other end, you may even decide to walk the short distance to the work place because you feel so good.

Throughout your day, you are liable to experience some restlessness and may well seek almost any excuse to wander around just to stop from becoming a tad irritable at having little to do, in the physical sense. To remain in one place for any length of time will not be a good idea at all.

The lack of just this basic exercise is unwelcome for you tend to feel almost frisky without knowing why and these little trips, no matter how frequent or pointless, maybe do help to work off an excess of physical well-being. Manual workers manage to get all of their tasks done and over with plenty of confidence and even ahead of their time which, if on an assembly line, could make them feel a little bored or even a little irritable.

Around the midday period, when they have to stop for a break, it is liable to be appreciated more for the chance to get a little exercise rather than still being machine or desk-bound. Eventually, the journey home will be approached with a tad more enthusiasm than usual. Once home, the slightest excuse to walk the dog, mow the lawn, redecorate or put some time in on the car will be welcomed with open arms.

If the individual is really athletic, he or she may prefer to spend some time playing football, tennis or other sport that they fancy. This is exactly what is needed when this physical positive phase with all of its feelings of a need to keep active is influencing you.

THE NEGATIVE PHASE

When the negative stage of this cycle influences the body, things are somewhat reversed. Waking up hurts, getting up is a real struggle and staying up even more so. When shaving, the men can and often do find it a trifle dodgy even with a fresh blade or a newly cleaned and sharpened electric shaver. He is likely to produce a cut or whatever and will probably forgo the aftershave. The ladies might wish they had never started their daily routine…

Breakfast will be a tad off-putting because, for most folk, a couple of sips of tea or coffee will suffice instead of food – of any kind. The walk to the station will be as equally regretted especially when fellow travellers seem to sort of almost race by while you struggle a step at a time. Once on board the train, you will do almost anything to get a seat and, once there, could almost drift off back to into the arms of Morpheus again.

On arrival at the main line station, the lift or escalator will be used gratefully and you are more than likely going to wait for a bus rather than face the short walk to work. On reaching your work-place, you make for the nearest chair for, having finally achieved this journey, you simply cannot yet face more action of any kind let alone the daily grind looming before you.

No matter how hard you try to ease off the morning load with coffee breaks, chats with fellow workers or sneaking off for a quiet smoke somewhere, the lunchtime break is most welcome because, no matter whatever else you may have been doing, you may now legitimately have a rest.

The act of actually going to get anything for your break will not attract at all and you will try somehow to make do with what you can get or ask someone else to do the job for you so that might even have a short nap. You will manage to get through the rest of your day somehow but the journey home won't be that welcome. Nevertheless, you finally get there.

Whatever plans you may have made for things you have thought of doing, you plant yourself in front of the box in the corner and there you will stay. The dog will have to walk itself, the grass must keep growing and everything else will just have to wait. Once back in your bed, actually trying to switch off may not be all that easy and although a deep sleep may overtake you eventually, come the morning, you will not feel as though you have had your fair share when you re-surface again.

Both of the foregoing descriptions are a tad over the top but they do illustrate how you might feel at such times – perhaps not quite so extreme as suggested but there are more occasions than you might think when we experience these good days or bad days. However, a close check will show that we do all have these kinds of times in cyclic periods more or less along the lines described.

When you come to examine such days a little more closely, this day or that day may well stand out, especially if it was when you pulled a muscle or made a serious mistake because you failed to take on board your abilities to carry out certain tasks. Silly little incidents and accidents like this often occur on critical days. It may seem strange, funny even, but these are the things that will happen at such times, that is, unless we first determine our capabilities for any given time.

THE CRITICAL DAY

When any of the cycles transit or change from one phase to the other, the day is known as a 'critical' day. Unfortunately, this label has appeared (or even hindered in some cases) to have popularised the whole concept of biorhythms perhaps more than anything else. Furthermore, and perhaps equally as unhelpfully, it has been proved that accidents are more likely to occur on a critical day than at any other time in any of the three main cycles.

Statistically, the probability of an incident or accident occurring on these days is very high, whether through lowered physical vitality, irrational emotional behaviour or inferior mental perception causing the subject to be more incident or accident prone.

Each rhythm has three critical days: at its beginning, the start of the cycle; at the half-way stage, when it changes from the positive to the negative phase; and at the end of the cycle, which, of course is also the commencement of the next positive phase.

If you look at the illustration you will see that a biogram for one month of 30 days has been created for the physical cycle which, in this example, starts on the first day of the month. The line marked '0' is normal but as this cycle (like the others) is continuous, there is no actual norm. The hand-drawn graph line is either above the line, below it or actually crossing it and the point at which the curve crosses the line, shows the critical day.

Straight away, therefore, we can tell that there are going to be three critical days this month. These will be on the 1st, 12th

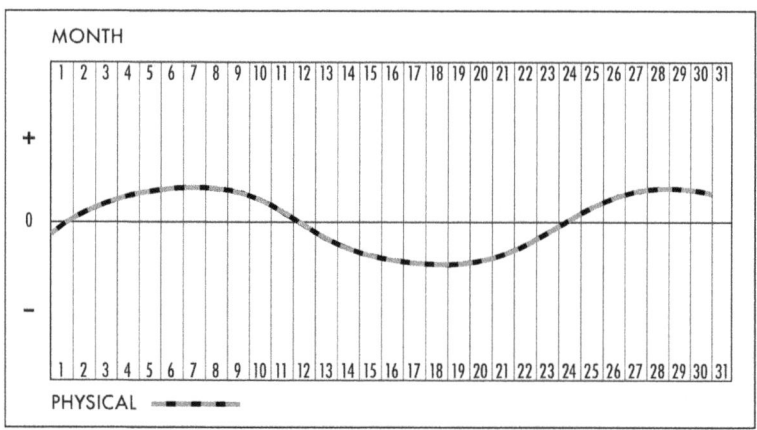

and 24th respectively, or when the curve begins to ascend into the positive stage on the first day; when it descends back over the line into the negative phase on the 12th and again when it returns to the line to end that cycle on the 24th to begin the next one.

Naming this point 'critical' is really quite wrong, mainly because nothing critical does actually take place. At such times, these changes in the cycle are simply a transition from one phase to another and might be better described as a turning point. However, it is a favourable or disturbing psychological moment whereby if anything is going to go wrong, it will be at this time, depending on the circumstances of the individual concerned.

THE POSITIVE PHASE

The physical rhythm starts on the first day of the month and rises into the positive phase, achieving its maximum extent at day seven: the 'mini-critical' day. Your physical abilities are at maximum potential on this seventh day peak and, if you are involved in any form of special physical activity, you ought to be able to give your best performance.

This is the one point of the positive phase where you should perform superbly well physically. However, you may just possibly overdo things and cause physical injury or discomfort in some way. In general, however, this is the best time to go all out for what you want, safe in the knowledge that you have everything going for you (in the physical sense, that is), provided you resist the temptation to overdo things.

THE NEGATIVE PHASE

In the negative phase, the lowest point of the cycle is reached on day eighteen. It is here that the rhythm begins to turn upward once again, eventually rising up into the positive phase, which it enters on the 24th day. This day is also the most negative part of the cycle, the trough, when this mini-critical period takes place. For most, it is the day of maximum lethargy – the subject feels as if he or she has little or no energy or inclination for anything.

Athletics at such a time are not to be recommended, save for routine practice. Often, it is on this negative mini-critical day that people tend to over-reach their potential by trying to do far more than they are capable of doing.

Work such as carpentry or gardening, trying to complete outstanding tasks that for some reason often fail to be finished on schedule but have to be concluded for all sorts of reasons, etc. These basically simple jobs are just the kind of thing that are so often unsuccessfully attempted at this stage. Now, if there is going to be an incident or accident caused by or through any physical incapacity, this is the day of highest probability.

MAKING ALLOWANCES

Again, it must be stressed that biorhythms in themselves do not have any cause and effect but are merely guidelines for timing events for the best results. There is no reason why you cannot perform all manner of physically strenuous tasks while in the negative stage or on critical or mini-critical days, provided that you allow for these particular conditions of the cycle.

For most sports people, especially the professionals who have to continually compete; it is their livelihood. Although most of them are fully aware of their capabilities backwards and even know of the cyclic behaviour patterns in their make-up, they have to allow for all or any temporary weaknesses and be hot to capitalise on them when they are on form.

Footballers, for example, are often reported that they seem to be 'off-form' because they miss the easy goals or other opportunities where they would ordinarily move in with their usual skills and win the moment. The same may be said of the cricketer who consistently bowls or bats for a few days in an appalling manner where he would normally have his hundred up or would have taken a wicket or two. Then there is the snooker player whose 'eye' is out where he would normally clear the table.

PHYSIOLOGICAL BASIS OF THE PHYSICAL RHYTHM

We are aware that the physical rhythm relates to basic muscle fibres. So, as everything in our bodies has a rhythm or a definite cyclic existence in some way it appears that everything to do with our physical capabilities materialises in the way we express our abilities on any given day. In other words, this is how we all tend to respond to our biological clocks.

There are a handful of folk who will be seen to vary from the norm and who seem to be always out of step with the rest of their immediate circle. The most obvious and clearest example of this will be observed in the phenomenon of 'day' or 'night' people, or the 'morning' and 'evening' folk.

The personal clocks of such folk are the same as everyone else, except that they always seem to be brighter or more physically active at different times of the day. Every individual responds to his personal 'inner' clock in exactly the same manner, but the timing may differ.

With most individuals, this can often be traced to the time of birth. Generally speaking, those who are born after noon seem to be 'night' people, that is, those who seem to come alive around 10 or 11 o'clock in the evening and stay this way through to the early hours. It would be rare for people born in the early hours to like the early hours in practice, but this is not an infallible issue. There are always exceptions to any rule but this might easily account for their personal foibles.

COMPATIBILITY

It would be a tad pointless trying to take on a round of golf if you are tired before you start because you will feel even more irritable and exhausted when you finish. In such cases, it would seem to be much more sensible to agree to a nine-hole exercise because you feel under par. Partners should be much more amenable under the circumstances because they ought to realise you are at least making an effort, even if they don't know why.

This is half the battle of successful relationships and goes a long way to improve any compatibility with those around you. Compromise, often such a dirty word to so many these days, should be effective when any situation is approached in such a fashion. Both of you want to enjoy yourselves, so to arrange the maximum pleasure possible in the right atmosphere at the right time, such a basic adjustment is far better than an outright refusal.

HEALTH

In the negative phase of the physical cycle there is almost always a strong health factor. You are much more prone to catch a chill or a cold or suffer indigestion as a result of inadequate or irregular meals that will upset your normal regular personal body functions as a result. During this phase, you are more susceptible to pain or, if you have an accident, you are likely to bleed more freely in the event of injury.

For example, should you have dental problems of any kind and you have to visit a dentist, try to make your appointment for the mid-afternoon period for this will be the best part of the day for when most people are resistant to this kind of discomfort. The worst time to experience dental pain is from around 03.00 hours through to about 09.00 in the morning.

Biorhythmically speaking, these two time periods are quite significant for any one suffering this type of pain. Of course, one does not 'allow' any kind of dental troubles to start at a particular time but the times given here are when you are your least or most susceptible to the pain involved.

Recovery from illness is often slower than usual at certain times of the day and, in some cases, even the night. This is so much so that doctors are beginning to time some operations to coincide with the plus phase of the patient's physical rhythm in order to facilitate recovery. Thus, pain becomes easier to cope with and the body feels in better fettle all round. Post-operative shock to the body is serious and, in some cases can kill, but this is considerably lessened if such time factors are taken into account.

Some patients on closely supervised courses of drugs may find that they are on a very strictly informed dosage and dosage times these days. It has been found that the old idea of 'three times a day after meals' can be very dangerous in certain circumstances. Doctors now know that what in some cases might be acceptable at 8 o'clock in the morning, can be positively lethal at 4 o'clock in the afternoon.

POWER SURGE

We can all remember those times when we have felt dreadfully low at around four or five o'clock in the afternoon. Times like this would have been accompanied with feelings of having to socialise whether we liked it or not because we were obliged to do so. Strangely, and a few hours later into the same evening, few would have realised that we, who felt totally out of it a few hours earlier, were now on top of the world and are simply not the same person.

Most normal people experience pulse variations during a 24-hour period and, where the average rate is around 72 beats per minute, in the evening it may be higher or lower by ten beats or even more. This makes a considerable difference to our physical responses. Generally speaking, the majority of people are at their lowest point in the early hours, even if they are 'night owls'. They bear little resemblance to the active person of twelve hours earlier or later when they were at their opposite level.

Another reason for such a change might occur during the actual twelve hours or so when we experience the critical day change period. It has been reported that some people feel a brief surge of power as their physical critical cycle changes from negative to positive. There are others who have suggested that they are aware of the switch from positive to negative when they feel a short period of extreme fatigue, lethargy or temporary indolence.

There are even a few people who have registered a critical day in their diary without knowing anything about biorhythms. They may have experienced severe indigestion or have eaten the wrong thing and just made do with a sandwich when what they really should have had was a proper meal and, of course, sufficient rest to go with it.

This is a major fault with those who drive long distances and tend to not take adequate rest away from the wheel. These are the folk who want to get the main task out of the way and then take time out for a meal and a rest.

NEGATIVE PHASE CARE

It must be fairly obvious by now that, even if you didn't know much about biorhythms before, you can now see that it makes sense to eat, drink and take adequate rest at regular intervals in order to allow the body to help maintain itself properly. If this is not carried out correctly, one can see how it might lead to an incident or accident occurring that could have been so easily avoided.

If your stamina levels are low on a physical critical day and meals are forgotten or you snack as an alternative, your mental perception might easily become less focussed. Quick reactions become dulled and a half-hearted response only is likely. In the extreme, this then becomes a possible difference between life and death. Excessive smoking as a substitute for eating a meal can cause a headache which, in the negative phase, leaves the body with little or no reserves on which to fall back on.

If your drinking habits, not necessarily alcohol, are allowed to get of hand, it will affect your sleeping levels. When in the negative phase and you fail to take the right amount of care, you will create an uneven set of energies in your body. Of course, none of us is perfect and it is not always possible to take the necessary rest and diet that we ought to do. Occasional lapses should remain that way – just occasional lapses, because they can and will create problems you don't want.

As long as you make sure you have regular meals, take moderate exercise and keep to routine habits, you will stay healthy when your biorhythms really so need you to support them. People who suffer with arthritis, asthma or rheumatism will find it so much easier to avoid such attacks by keeping an eye on their physical cycle; especially if or when uncertain weather conditions are predicted. The early hours of the day are when people are most susceptible to such attacks, while the mid-afternoon period is best for them to indulge in light exercise, should they feel the need to do so.

Those of you with blood pressure or heart conditions should avoid trying to drive for too long when the physical rhythm is adverse. In these conditions, one should never drive on an empty stomach because the blood sugar levels may be lowered more than the body may be able to withstand and that can lead to them being accident-prone.

READING THE SIGNS

Should you be aware of the 'condition' your physical cycle is in, this will help to ease some of the tensions of any normal day as they build up. When you know your potential is below par, it is always half the battle, for it serves to help read the danger signs and, of course, make any adjustments in plenty of time.

Driving can be a little more troublesome at such times and even if you are not the initial cause of an accident, you must remember that your reactions are poorer on critical days, no matter which way the cycle is heading.

You would do well to also remember, those who say they sense that small surge of power on negative to positive changeover days often speak of a tremendous feeling of well-being and physical bonhomie. It is more likely that they have lulled themselves into a false sense of security and that their abilities and judgment are liable to be faulty. Long driving spells on a critical day takes its toll because you probably haven't noticed how much energy you use at such times. On long distance journeys it is surprising how much the body moves when seated freely. The introduction of the seat belt laws helps to restrict body movement and a lot of energy is conserved that might otherwise be frittered away.

Educating our minds to our abilities as they are and not as we think they might be is not that easy. Despite an occasional lazy streak we do sometimes tend to overdo things if out of the ordinary tasks need to be performed. These are the occasions when accidents are likely to happen.

We become so caught up with other matters we tend not to notice (or choose to ignore) all those little aches and pains and put them down to unaccustomed physical activity. We are right, but we forget that these are part of the body's natural early-warning system.

Swimming is a good example. It is a pastime that really does take far more out of us than we fully appreciate. On critical days, we should be very careful indeed; not just because cramp may set in and temporarily cripple us, but because of the blind panic that often drowns the victim in such circumstances.

The two are inextricably linked: if we had not overdone the one, we may not experience the other extreme. There are more cases of drowning on double critical days, that is, the physical and emotional or physical and intellectual days, than at any other time. Perhaps a little more thought here might not have seen the event end in tragedy.

OVERSTEPPING THE LIMIT

These days far too many of us live on nervous energy and dismiss the physical limits we think we can and so often do ignore. However, sooner or later, the time of reckoning

THE PHYSICAL CYCLE

sneaks up on us all. Had we monitored our physical cycle less indifferently, we might have eased much unnecessary stress and strain that we can all do without.

Stress is a killer, and these are stressful times. In simple terms, stress often comes about because we fail to realise what or how we are faring or whatever it is we are doing, where we obviously cannot see the wood for the trees. For most of us, our present way of life, especially in our towns and cities, involves a lot of stress. When the bus or train is cancelled, or, if it is running late, when it does arrive, you find that you are unable to board because it is full.

The boss might ask of you more than you can reasonably be expected to give but you either cannot or will not say anything. Stress may also be created when friends who ask for help get shirty when you say no because you can't, won't or don't feel up to it. When you ask somebody to do you a favour and they refuse, a little more stress still comes into the act. It is at times like this when you really must learn to monitor your physical well-being. If your physical biorhythm is in the negative phase, ease back as much as you can. When in the positive stage, try not to overdo things. Remember, there are many ways in which your physical rhythm alone can be used to your best advantage.

You don't have to stop enjoying activities, because this rhythm is in its negative phase for about ten days or so or is at a critical point. All you need to do is lessen the pressures you feel building up and then take steps to compensate the body for its lack or over-abundance of energy.

Once you enter into the swing of things and start to enjoy this new style of routine, it will soon become second nature to use biorhythms more intelligently. Preparation for negative phases can be taken at a much steadier pace than before and you will find that life will become far more manageable. Those little extra efforts you make for critical and mini-critical days soon become a way of life. And during the positive periods you can make the most of your abilities as you see fit.

There will be some occasions when you will not be able to plan ahead and make the simple adjustments you would like, but if you have your bio-chart to hand, at least you will know just how far you can safely go.

In itself, that must surely be reward enough.

CHAPTER 4

THE EMOTIONAL CYCLE

This rhythm lasts for 28 days and, although more commonly called the emotional cycle, it is also widely recognised as the sensitivity rhythm. It is concerned mainly with our moods, sensitivity and social ability and, while it is the easiest of all the rhythms to chart, it is also perhaps the most difficult of the three with which we have to contend. One of the most helpful associations is that the day upon which you experience a critical day, coincides with the day that you were born. Thus, if you were born on a Sunday, every other Sunday will be a critical day. We will deal with this in more detail later.

Unfortunately, and for a variety of reasons this rhythm is often the most misunderstood.

There have been many claims of links with astrology here because of the length of the cycle which, up to a point, may seem to coincide with lunar phasing. Such a claim, while vague and quite unsupported, is completely invalid. The suggestion that there are also links with the female menstruation cycle because the two may coincide for a while, also comes to nothing when they are compared. While the emotional cycle never varies, the female rhythm can and does.

THE EMOTIONAL POSITIVE PHASE

This cycle which appears be ruled rather largely by and through the nervous system has been described as a manifestation of the cells that seem to influence the feminine side of our nature whether or not we ourselves are male or female.

The first part of this rhythm, the positive or plus phase is when we are our normal cheerful, optimistic and responsive selves. The first fourteen days are favourable for just about all of our creative interests, whether it might be a simple friendship, a deep romance or the usual socially co-operative side of our nature.

Perhaps one of the most important and active part of our lives, that of co-ordination, plays a most active role in this cycle. It is very important in and to our nervous system that we need to 'feel' that things are right before any of these issues can be considered. In the negative phase of this cycle, co-ordination is so often markedly absent.

By the eighth day of the positive phase, most individuals tend to experience a strong sense of well-being. This is when our sociability peaks and it is at this point in the cycle that the emotional sensitivity is at its highest level. However, on this so-called mini-critical day, many people appear to become over-confident and overdo things because of the way they feel.

After this point, the rhythm curves down towards the critical day halfway through the cycle. The general performance of people is still acceptable and quite good but it is starting to lose its edge.

EMOTIONAL CRITICAL DAYS

Like the physical cycle, the emotional rhythm starts off with a critical day, has its transition day from positive to negative fourteen days later and ends on the third critical day, fourteen days after that. It, too, has mini-critical days with the first one falling on the 8th day in the positive phase and on the 22nd day in the negative stage.

THE EMOTIONAL CYCLE

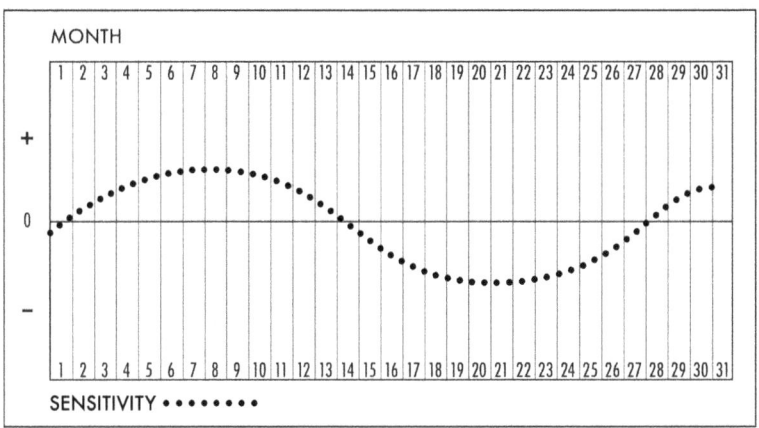

If you look at the illustration you will see that a biogram for one month of thirty days has been created for the emotional cycle which, in this example, starts on the first day of the month. The line marked '0' is normal but as this cycle (like the others) is continuous, there is no actual norm. The hand drawn graph line is either above the line, below it or actually crossing it and the point at which the curve crosses the line shows the critical day.

Straight away, therefore, we can tell that there are going to be three critical days this month. These will be on the 1st, 14th and 28th respectively, or when the curve begins to ascend into the positive stage on the first day; when it descends back over the line into the negative phase on the 14th and again when it returns to the line to end that cycle on the 28th to begin the next one.

There is one very useful effect that comes with this particular cycle. Because it is of a steady 28 day nature, it means that if, for example, you were born on a Sunday, then each alternate Sunday would be a critical day. In addition, every Sunday would mark a day whereby all of your emotional peaks and troughs in the cycle with their associated behaviour patterns will also occur. For some, this may account for the way many of us lay claim to having a 'favourite day' idea. Not everybody appreciates this association but it is rather helpful when assessing which will be (are or were) your good days or bad days.

On an emotional critical day, you are at your most vulnerable to a rather wide selection of emotional reactions, irrespective of which way the rhythm may be travelling at the time. Irritability, insensitivity or even irrationality will probably be the most likely responses shown at such times. Any different environmental situation will not create much in the way of a problem, although the environment or any out of the ordinary conditions should normally be taken into account.

During the emotional critical day, even the calmest of people have been known to explode at a crucial moment if or when things do not go their way. Conversely, the most volatile have been known to pass through this period without raising an eyebrow. As the rhythm appears to control everything to do with our emotional response at all levels, it follows that it must take on an added importance in our relationships. This is not to mention potential incident or accident situations or anything else that needs our drive and enthusiasm to be working at full strength in our favour.

The success of a party or any other type of get-together does become somewhat lowered on day 22 of this cycle. This would be especially so if it also coincided with a physical negative stage and or an intellectual critical day. Nevertheless, such an adverse time in these cycles is to be on the cards, as long as your recognise the limitations, the event may still take place as long as you make an the effort and attempt to remain on even keel.

On an emotional critical day, almost anything can happen if any kind of stress is generated through emotive issues. Of these three rhythms, this cycle is the most prone to error, incidents and accidents. Your thinking will be coloured by your emotional reactions to what is going on around you.

You may start the day well but if the slightest thing upsets you, then you will exhibit an ultra-touchy and quite over-sensitive mood often without realising it. For example, should you be out driving and are overtaken by another vehicle, you might well be tempted to chase after it and re-overtake the other driver – if nothing else, just to show that you can. It may sounds silly and dramatic, but thousands of us are prone to do such things and these reactions have been recorded for emotionally critical days.

Another reaction that you may show is when you and your partner have been planning to go out for the evening and have been looking forward to the event throughout the day. However, your partner might delay or criticise you in some large or small way. Now, no matter how well-meaning such an action may be, you are liable to over-react. You may sulk, refuse to go or start a row probably quite unintentionally.

In another environment, a small almost unnoticed event might happen and if you are in charge you might use your authority to dismiss the person responsible. When or where others may interpret this as a mere triviality, to you in your present mood it appears as a most heinous offence.

THE NEGATIVE PHASE

When this rhythm turns into the negative phase, people become less co-operative generally. They will also exhibit moodiness, sensitivity and can be touchy beyond belief in some cases.

Some folk become depressed and fixated with issues that may not ordinarily worry them. They tend to feel the world owes them a living or that people seem to be 'against' them for some reason. Those who have to associate closely with others when in this phase are liable to notice these changes the most – probably because they have become quite used to their funny little ways.

Another effect is that people in this stage of the cycle may well become demon-shoppers. They find fault with everyone and everything from the assistant in the store to the decor of the shop. They make a point of checking their change so deliberately that the cashier feels that they are insulting not only their intelligence but also their feelings.

Curiously, few if any people realise their behaviour patterns are having this effect on other folk. When in the negative stage of this cycle, especially on the 22nd day or the nadir of the cycle, everything and everyone becomes their enemy. They have a completely negative outlook on everything and everybody with moods that can be quite extreme. However, as the cycle begins to move slowly toward the next critical day, life appears to become more bearable – in their eyes. When the critical day arrives, they will probably seem to show a tad more humour than usual. There may be a show of over-confidence and a desire to take on additional responsibility – usually a lot more than they can really handle.

As a rule, the normal change-over period for the physical cycle is around 24 hours. However, at least 48 hours should be allowed for the emotional cycle. This serves to allow plenty of time in which to clear away any possible lapses in behaviour patterns. It would be a good idea to forgo driving if at all possible. As the danger of an incident or an accident can loom large at such times, it would be a good idea to not put them into any situation where an unnecessary risk can be avoided.

As most of us tend to experience something along the lines of these imbalances because of what we do, where we are or whatever, we should not close down until the time is over. In some countries this is more or less what does happen. In parts of Japan, some drivers are asked to work indoors for the duration of a critical day or, should they drive anywhere, they are asked to show a small flag that tells everyone of their current biorhythmic state.

In some of the Japanese towns and cities where biorhythms are almost a way of life, some of the taxi-drivers have such a fanatical enthusiasm for such events that it can be a fairly regular sight to see the flags flying from their cars.

THE QUESTION OF FREE WILL

Arguments can be used to prove some of the claims regarding our potential behavioural patterns but how do we try to explain such events that are basically free will? Even if nothing happens, and may never do so in some cases, our biorhythms are a reliable guide for avoiding possible troubles. It shouldn't be blindly accepted as a certainty that, just because we will shortly have a critical day, we must do this or that.

We usually choose our way of life to conform to and with our surroundings, but this may not always be possible. The con-man, business genius, artist, hero or heroine all have their own level of sufficient free will to choose their actions in the way they want. However, the majority of us feel it better to conform by seeking and settling for the best niche in society and staying there. The only time we might move out this environment is when the urge to do so calls us or by invitation.

We are at our most vulnerable in defence of our niche when we feel above or below the norm and are tempted to stray away from the path we have selected for ourselves. We all feel comfortable when we fit in with everything round us although there are a few folk who tend (prefer?) to stay out in the cold a tad longer than most. In competitive events, the most natural thing is to want (need?) to win. How we achieve this is reflected in our behaviour patterns.

Of course, there is always the regular competitive type who must win and uses everything in his or her power to do so but there is also the rank outsider who is considered to not have a chance. The emotional rhythm in the positive phase will favour both contenders and they should share equal chances at the starting line – but it is the performance that counts. Entertainers perform better when their cycle is in the positive stage. Those little nuances we use to express ourselves more effectively are of especial importance to a comedian when he or she practises their art.

USING THE POSITIVE STAGE

To contribute to any kind of teamwork requires a little acting ability, commitment and concentration. One also has to put to one side or disguise any preferences they may have. In business, police work, sport, selling or advertising, it is necessary to have these abilities and to be able to handle a certain amount of sublimation of your personal needs and desires if you are to achieve the aim. The positive stage of the emotional cycle is almost always the best time to make this kind of an effort. Even television newsreaders or programme presenters are less likely to fluff their lines at such a time and manage to stay on an even keel.

When or if you decide to propose to your current partner, it would be most wise to establish your mutual biorhythm status for the best results. And here there are a wide variety of surprises, for it has been found that many really happy couples often have a total variance in their respective rhythms which will be dealt with more fully in the chapter on compatibilities.

However, if you are about to propose, at the very least ensure that your emotional cycle is in its positive phase. Whatever the response, you will be better able to handle the results of your proposal then. If you are planning any large-scale business ventures, do so in the positive stage of this rhythm. If nothing else, this will help you to put over the idea and show the necessary enthusiasm for others to follow.

To be successful in such matters, you must be on the ball, ready to cope with any adverse situations and be able to handle question and answer sessions positively.

When the physical cycle is in the positive stage, you can happily take part in most sporting activities and fully enjoy the experience. However, if the physical or emotional phase is negative, all you have to do is remember your physical ability for the day in question and not overdo anything.

ALLOWING FOR THE NEGATIVE PHASE

When you are in the negative stage there is no real reason why you may not take part in any activity as long as you allow for your possible limitations of the moment as indicated by your chart. If you allow for a 48 hour period here for this critical time you can join in just about anything you like – even if there is an element of danger involved. Just bear in mind your limitations if you do.

Of course, if you want to kill yourself then go ahead, for there are many open air events you can enjoy as a competitor that you ought to avoid like the plague at such times because you will be error prone. Horse trials, motor car or motor cycle sport, diving and swimming are all fraught with danger for anyone at the wrong time. Of course the other problem here is that you could take someone else with you and, perhaps, be responsible for their demise as a result of your inability to cope. And this is where knowing the positions of the cycles of someone else is so useful.

BIORHYTHMIC PRE-KNOWLEDGE OF OTHERS

Biorhythms do not predict the outcome of an event but they do show the potential at your disposal. How you use this information is entirely up to you. The principal advantage of the knowledge of your biorhythmic state allows you to know your particular abilities for the activity in question. So, what biorhythms must do for you they must also do for everyone else and this is where the really astute types truly come into their own.

One sales manager had the biorhythm charts for his entire sales force prepared along with their main buyers. With some clever juggling here and some careful timing there, the sales graphs eventually went through the roof. Some of the new 'partnerships' that were 'created' had an almost immediate positive effect. The advantage of being aware of another person's abilities allowed the members of these new teams to capitalise positively on this knowledge.

This was not unfair, it was using biorhythms intelligently to gain more out of life – and not only did this scheme work for this man it is also open to everyone else to do the same.

If you have high blood pressure, you have a need to avoid deliberately taking risks on an emotionally critical day. The sensible person will have his or her chart prepared and then be ready to curb their tongue should a slip affect business relationships in important policy matters. People in this state should concentrate on the smaller issues, tidy up loose ends and relax a little more when they realise that their concentration may not be so easy.

When you lack perception but can improve your performance by as much as 50% or more, then it is time you learned to re-organise your affairs so that they always favour you. Perhaps one of the worst possible places to be is in the office where and when the annual Christmas party takes place, for this so often shows people at their worst.

If you are easily embarrassed and it seems as if it will not be a good day for you then you have two choices. Make a reasonable excuse and not go, but this may be wrongly misinterpreted by those who matter. So, attend the event but keep a low profile and just slip away at the earliest opportunity. The sudden freedom involved at such gatherings and often before the alcohol kicks in frequently shows people exhibiting almost perfect biorhythmic responses. If you were to check individual charts prior to such times it might prove to be more useful and ensure that all get the best from the event.

Naturally, not everyone's biorhythms will be ideally phased at the same time, but a careful and considerate host will ensure no one gets left out of the fun entirely. We often find that we can get along with certain people even when our biorhythms indicate that we should not be in company at all.

Emotional compatibility and sensitivity to atmosphere requires astute handling. A careless word here or a wrong deed there can prove very embarrassing but, more to the point, it is likely to stay in the memory of other folk for longer than you think.

The simplest advice is to remember what could happen and behave accordingly. You are then well on the way to automatically correct behaviour in your relationships. These positive patterns are always noticed by those who matter. It is at times like this when such folk are likely to be singled out for promotion much earlier than may be reasonably expected. Others may be given a project they may not ordinarily have thought they could handle – and so on.

The people who work in employment agencies often seem to exhibit 'attitudes' toward people out of work for a variety of reasons. On occasions, they seem suited to what they do while at others they appear to be completely out of place. Their best times for such duties should be (need to be might be a better term) assessed by a biorhythmic check so that other tasks could be quite easily handled on a temporary basis on their more inauspicious days.

Similarly, teachers whose cycles are not good for announcing instructions clearly might better use their time for setting or correcting written work. If the class plays up, any loss of face would be more easily averted. The general discipline level in the school might well eventually improve as result. There is little worse than a teacher who displays his or her temper or who becomes involved in a slanging match with a pupil.

This collection of ideas reflects just a few of the lessons we ought to take on board simply by keeping a weather eye on the emotional rhythm alone. When we do this sort of thing and involve all three rhythms together, it almost always improves people's performance. Those who remain on an even keel in times of adversity do get noticed and do receive the right rewards for their positive actions. When this also helps our relationship with other folk as well, there can be no end to what we can achieve – and none of us can live without others.

CHAPTER 5

THE INTELLECTUAL CYCLE

This, the third cycle in our investigations suggests a certain amount of control in and around all of our intellectual responses. Our powers of reason, judgment, perception and just plain old fashioned common sense seem also to be the principal arenas of activity.

The positive phase, as with each of the other cycles, begins with a critical day and serves to accentuate each of these activities mainly to the good. You shine mentally, your powers of observation are at their best and simple mental problems are dealt with so readily and easily you often complete a task without realising it.

Intellectually, you feel in fine fettle and want to exercise what you think is your under-employed state of mind. There might even be a tendency to take part in simple, light hearted calculations from your observations or you may test your memory with mental games just for the sheer pleasure of flexing the mind. Crossword puzzle enthusiasts will be in their element at such times.

So, a book of reasonably easy puzzles of any kind at this stage of your cycle is highly recommended because, when you feel your mental processes need to be exercised, you could become bored quite quickly and may even stagnate. Any active mind that is left to its own devices may well create a problem at just about any level. People in this stage are likely to make cutting, hurtful or sarcastic remarks. Even a justifiable criticism that would have been better left alone can quickly spoil an otherwise good relationship if incorrectly phrased.

THE POSITIVE INTELLECTUAL PHASE

It is doubtful whether we ever use our brains to full capacity and this rhythm of thirty-three days, if not properly understood and properly used, will almost certainly create problems with what is, after all, your most valuable asset.

The mind is a funny thing for, the more it is used, the better it flourishes. It is rather like a car engine in that the more you use it (and preferably correctly), the more efficiently it will serve you. If you continue to make short journeys on a regular basis, sooner or later your car will need to be serviced that little bit earlier. The same goes with your brain or the mind. The more you flex your mental muscles the better it will serve you.

So, in the positive phase of this cycle, the best thing to do is to keep the mind as stimulated as you can. Students find that their mind will absorb more information in an half hour of study during this positive phase than they can achieve in a whole day when their intellectual cycle is in its negative stage. All types of creative pursuits yield far better results, ideas flow more fluently and perception is at its highest point.

All the mental senses are much more acute and responsive at a much higher level than normal. All forms of debate and discussion proceed in your favour, unless other people are in the same state, in which case this really will be a meeting of minds. Your ego is strong, conversation will flourish and you get along swimmingly with all around you. Because

THE INTELLECTUAL CYCLE

your perceptivity is at such a high level, within the space of an hour or so a whole host of subjects can be covered over after-dinner brandy, coffee and cigars. Just how many may well surprise you.

Ambitious folk, those with definite aims in life and those who need to impress people who matter would do well to wait for this cycle to be in its positive phase and, preferably at around day nine when they are at the mini-critical stage of this rhythm. Your powers of concentration, perception and ability to reason things through quickly (and correctly) will have that little extra edge and power which may well be apparent to any observer. Should you have to attend a meeting of any kind, your grasp of what is happening will be noted by the boss, his or her managers and anyone else looking for people to position in the right place for the right reasons.

The ability to plan events will come almost as a second nature. Details that matter will not be forgotten especially those that might ordinarily escape the notice of others less perceptive at the time. When money troubles need to be properly sorted out, who better than you and your ability to create and keep to a budget which will take care of everything.

Up to a point, this is not a bad time to begin a new job. New routines are remembered so much easier and the many fresh faces will be easier to recognise. All these matters will be handled easily and masterfully almost as if you had always been there. The difficult side of any social problems will come to you more easily because your mental capacity and processes will work so well. You will have all the time in the world to get all the facts straight, remembered and handled so proficiently.

It would also be rather helpful if your emotional biorhythm was also in a positive phase, for this will soften the hard business approach and allow you to present less pressure so often needed for the first few days in any new job.

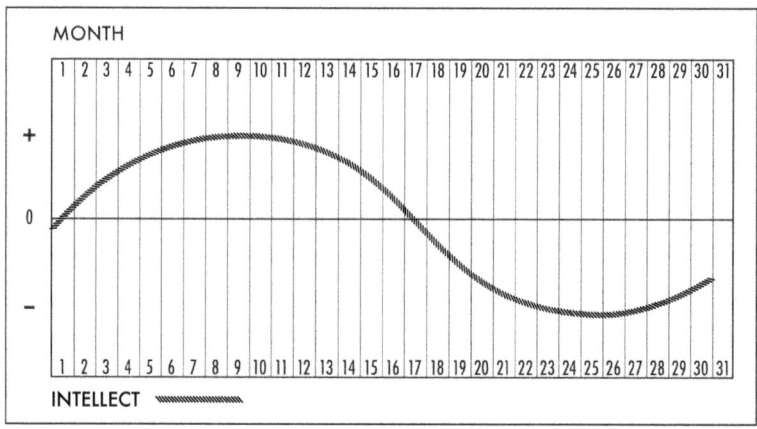

If you look at the illustration you will see that a biogram for one month of 30 days has been created for the intellectual cycle which, in this example, starts on the first day of the month. The line marked '0' is normal but as this cycle (like the others) is continuous, there is no actual norm. The hand drawn graph line is either above the line, below it or actually crossing it and the point at which the curve crosses the line shows the critical day.

Straight away, therefore, we can tell that there are going to be only two critical days this month. These will be on the 1st and the 17th respectively, or when the curve begins to ascend into the positive stage on the first day and when it descends back over the line into the negative phase on the 17th. As the rhythm is of 33 days duration, there can only be two critical days in any month.

INTELLECTUAL CRITICAL DAYS

On a day like this your perception becomes greatly impaired, intelligence becomes muddled and you may well feel a tad fuzzy or muddled. As the day moves on, it might well become harder for you to more properly express yourself. On a critical day in this cycle, forgo any calls on decision making or anything that needs good judgment and common sense. On top of all this, your memory will not be that reliable either. Travel matters could also be problematic if in unfamiliar territory.

The intellectual critical day often has a slightly longer effect than that of the physical cycle. So, as with the emotional rhythm, it would be a wise person who allows at least 48 hours before you can consider yourself really free of the effects.

Thus, should you be approaching a period where you have important meetings scheduled or other things that will require you to make and take decisions that could affect your immediate or distant future and you are nearing an intellectual critical day, it would be a wise move to postpone the issue. Because of the way we live these days, it may not always be an easy matter to postpone. So, if this should be the case, you must remember that you are almost certainly going to be error-prone at a time when you can least afford it.

Of course, you may think that nothing may go wrong and that you will probably sail through it all. And that is what is meant by being error prone – you might have forgotten an important point, or didn't go back over what you have said or done to check for errors or omissions. On days like these, you must take your time. You won't want to look 'slow' in the eyes of people who matter but, if you have made an error or two, at least you will have found it before any real damage has been done.

If you are a pay clerk and unwittingly credit an employee with more than he or she should have received, the chances of getting the money back may be difficult. But if you double checked your work in time and found that you have made a mistake, it ought to be relatively easy to correct once you have found out who was wrongly paid.

When in a position like this, where you are held responsible for irregularities in your cash dealings, such an error could cost you dearly. Your ability, honesty, integrity and reputation all come under scrutiny when all you did was make a simple error that anyone else could have made in similar circumstances.

THE NEGATIVE PHASE

When the cycle moves into its negative phase, your mental abilities slow down, perception is hard, your acuity is dulled and you will probably find it hard to put together a three piece jigsaw puzzle. Your level of concentration just goes straight out of the window and trying to read a book is a waste of time altogether. And while you are at it, do stay away from your computer or you may quite innocently wipe out the memory. Even the most basic task can seem like hard work at such times.

Not everyone suffers like this. Many people rarely feel anything is wrong and may not exhibit any problems at such times. It does happen to a rare few though. For example, a college teacher who continually flexes his or her mental muscles might only exhibit a slight difference when this cycle moves into the negative phase.

A fluffed line here or a short pause there while the memory appears to be faulty all of a sudden may well coincide on or about day 24 or 25 when we all experience a mini-critical day in the negative stage of this rhythm. At such times, we are likely to inadvertently address someone by their wrong name or title.

Sportsmen are called on to live a much more physical life than the average person and it was also once thought that these people did not need to use their mental processes half as much as a teacher or someone in a similar profession

THE INTELLECTUAL CYCLE

might. These days this type of reasoning has to be called into question. All sport demands a lot of hard concentration and requires all its competitors to be very much in the right frame of mind.

For example, many tennis players are taught to balance their biorhythms on a regular basis. A low physical cycle may be cleverly used with the positive intellectual cycle to avoid being unnecessarily distracted. Because tennis people have to rely on themselves and their own skills to survive they can and do often work wonders when they have their personal biorhythm calendars to which they may refer.

People who work as editors as well as writers and authors have to rely on their intellectual ability and prowess to produce good work all the time. Perhaps there are a few better tasks than here to introduce the role biorhythms play in people's lives.

If anything has changed over the past 30 years or so, the tasks of an editor certainly has. While many still actually work on an actual manuscript, most of them now check and edit material on a computer screen. He or she has to be especially careful in their critical periods because mistakes can cost a small fortune with many of them.

Several editors of my acquaintance have had their biorhythm charts compiled to offset any potential problems at such times. Without exception, they all say that they feel the workload is now so much easier.

A writer's life has eased a lot in comparison for much of what they write is now created on a computer screen and, what with all the help word processors offer these days, it is far better than typing things out only to find an error on the last line when the work is checked.

The same goes for authors as well. My very first book compiled in 1974 had to be written in long hand first and then typed for submission afterwards. It was a long and hard period not just for me but also for those had to check it all later. All I have to do these days is be aware of my 'off' times and go and do something else.

Sometimes, however, this is not always possible. Editing is a hard job at the best of times. Even at the peak of my abilities (biorhythmically speaking) mistakes can still occur but they are found more easily. The real secret of editing is to read out loud to yourself what is actually written and **not** what you think has been written (try reading what is actually there out loud to yourself). Once that task has been mastered the rest is easy.

Our lives have speeded up somewhat considerably in the last 20 to 30 or so years and so also has the need to be able to cope with it all. Biorhythms were never more useful than they are now. No matter what job you think of or what activity comes to mind, all could be better handled when you know what your own abilities and limitations are and that is why more and more people use them.

As a rule, the opinion of most biorhythm exponents is that the second half of the intellectual rhythm, the negative phase, should be used for all kinds of review work where possible. Just about anything new is better tackled during the intellectual positive stage, for that is when most actors and actresses have found it so much easier to work their way through new scripts. Their mind is much more perceptive and can handle anything new reasonably well.

In the negative phase, it really doesn't want to have to tackle any new material. Their mind is ticking over gently – an ideal time for appraising information or material already gathered.

Curiously, crime detection often peaks in this phase. An investigating police officer, especially one with many years under his or her belt has to review their work and that of others over and over again. They have to repeatedly piece together everything to do with a case so many times and the painstaking care with which they have to do this is well-known. If they are to get an inspiration or a lead from the facts as they are at the time, it will usually be when they are in the negative stage of the intellectual cycle. On top of this, it is always helpful if they delay the arrest of their main suspect until when that worthy adversary is experiencing their intellectually critical day.

This may not always be possible, so the police have to be absolutely sure of their facts before moving in. This is such a good idea because we so often hear of cases being lost because of a legal technicality in the suspect's favour. Research on this point might throw up some interesting facts. At present, the only information we have to hand is that crime occurs 4.7% times more frequently on intellectually critical days than on positive ones.

Serious crimes, such as murder, rape, kidnapping or armed robbery take place most often when the subject is in the positive phase of the physical cycle with the other two cycles in negative phase. This is often a time when so many villains seem so capable of great violence. Unfortunately, we can only view crime problems in retrospect. A quick glance through police records supports this theory, although there isn't enough information available to confirm it beyond all reasonable doubt.

Many politicians of all standings are often quite susceptible to fluctuations in their intellectual rhythm. So much in the public eye at all times, they are acutely aware that they are public figures and tend to behave quite well most of the time. However, if they are going to make a mistake, it will almost always be on a critical day, usually in the intellectual cycle, more than at any other time.

Politics may be said to be a more mentally-orientated way of life as well as being rather taxing. But so many politicians have put their feet well and truly in it at many inopportune moments that biorhythms have proven their worth – from the observer's point of view, of course.

AWARENESS OF POTENTIAL

Intellectual mini-critical days occur on day 9 in the positive phase and day 26 in the negative stage, which suggests the amount of ability the subject is likely to exhibit. In the plus stage, mistakes or over confidence often occur, almost as if the person concerned has neglected to do his or her homework. However, there is also a likelihood of the subject showing one or two brilliant streaks of originality on occasion.

The opposite is true in the negative stage. It almost seems as if the mind cannot cope with any situation and what mistakes are made are often real howlers. These are extreme examples, of course, but they serve to illustrate the way in which biorhythms can be employed as guidelines for living.

We do not suggest people cannot live without a biorhythm chart to hand at all times or that accidents tend to occur on critical days because such incidents can and do happen at other times. However, by now, the reader must be aware that it has to be to their advantage to be as aware as possible of their personal limitations before they attempt anything new.

After all, it has been statistically proved that we are more likely to survive incidents and accidents when our physical and intellectual cycles are positive and our emotional rhythm is negative than at any other time. The intellectual cycle is the least studied of the three main rhythms, partly because research into the physical side of biorhythms seems to be connected with the physical rhythm as well as the emotional cycle. Nevertheless, the intellectual rhythm should be given the same importance as the other two because life can so often be a series of logical – or illogical – steps.

THE INTELLECTUAL CYCLE

BIORHYTHMS – A KEY TO SUCCESS

Just about all that you do has to do with your social obligations. When you stop and think seriously about it all, it is because you feel the need to fit in and not to cause too many waves. We all need to be an integral part of the society level(s) in which we either choose or have to exist. In simple terms, this is often called survival. Everybody around you, no matter what their standing in your association obeys the same impulses and observe the same rigorous codes of behaviour that you do.

Admittedly, although each of us interprets our way of life in our personal and individual style, some people will stand out more but not necessarily better than others. Those who have given up are people like the down-and-outs or the other unfortunates who have experienced more than they could handle in their once normal way of life and gave up the struggle. People who really stand out these days are those who seem to seize each opportunity as it arises and somehow manage to turn it to their advantage.

Who is to say they have not used their brains to achieve their positions which you may envy? Many prefer to opt for the argument that these people got where they are because their faces fitted or because they had all the right contacts in all the right places at the right time and that ability had little to do with their success. Up to a point, this is not an unreasonable supposition where some folk are concerned, yet some of them had to have had an ability that got them noticed in the first place. That is, an ability to think things through, reason and make decisions based on a predetermined course or by following their natural desires.

The naturally ambitious always succeed because they use what they have to their advantage – theirs and that of everyone else around them as well. The intelligent use of biorhythms could have you up there with them vying for the same things on equal terms.

Of course, biorhythms do not give you any special or original ability to succeed, for that is not possible. But what abilities you do have can be enhanced by timing all of your opportunities to the best possible advantage. We all want to succeed and, when they are used intelligently, your biorhythms will help you along the all-important road to success.

CHAPTER 6

CALCULATIONS

One of the principal problems with biorhythms has always been in the way they are (or have to be) worked out without the use of a calculator or a computer. However, since the middle 1970's there have been quite a few alternative methods with which one may arrive at the various phases, stages and critical days.

Here in the UK, few people attempted to pursue the study, partly because of how to calculate them properly. When I wrote and created the first book on the subject in this country in 1980, this was very much on my mind. After just over ten years study, the effort was well worthwhile and the work was a success. I have discussed all the different ways one can use but have kept the whole system as basically simple as I can.

The methods have included the use of specialised calculators that will complete these tasks for you in a matter of moments. Unfortunately, for a long while, most of these were limited to work from January 01 1901 through to December 31 1999. There were once several of these 'dedicated' calculators on the market all of which were more or less variations on a theme. Each in their own way produced the figures for the day in question at the touch of a button or two. However, they were limited to work for any date but only within the last century.

However, there are now many different computer programs specifically designed that make the whole task so much easier these days, even for those who do not have trouble working out these things. In addition, there are several books that have now been published which have included various ways of arriving at the right date to those that created predetermined codes. All you had to do was look up your personal information in the tables provided. There are even a couple authors who have published books with a 100 year set of biorhythms to save you the time.

Before or after the century date change of the current century and the 18th over the 19th you had to rely on your own abilities with manual arithmetic. While not a difficult task, it was (and, quite frankly, still is) a long-winded affair. Now that we are well into the early part of the 21st century, computer programs proliferate everywhere and there are even applications you can use on your mobile phone. With many of these applications, short interpretations for the day in question are presented. However, they are incredibly varied with some actually contradicting each other.

With most computer programs, one can calculate dates and days across the centuries because they have been programmed to allow for this as well as to note the change from the Julian calendar system to the present Gregorian one that most countries use today. Nevertheless, it would be wise to note that here in the UK we changed over from the old (Julian calendar) to the one we use today in September 1752 – the Gregorian calendar.

In the early days, you were asked to apply for your personal biograms that were created in slightly differing formats. For a small cash layout you could obtain a computer print-out for a month, three months, a year or even longer. Hand-drawn biograms were and still are created for a month, three months, six months, a one-year period or more and in some places such a service is still available.

People may also apply to have their biorhythmic state charted in retrospect for a specific day or period in their past life or for a future event. Many folk might also write and ask for the state of a famous or infamous personality from the past or present. There was, and still is no general conformity in the way these are presented.

You may also apply to have your own compatibility with that of other people who may be close to you or, perhaps, for someone else for whatever reason, as described elsewhere in this book.

STYLE OF PRESENTATION

Visually, the easiest style to understand is the generally acceptable small card style with the agreed colour code where the physical cycle should always be drawn in red, the emotional cycle presented in blue and the intellectual cycle written in green ink. However, do be careful for this system is not always used and, in some cases if you are not ready for such things, life can become a tad difficult here.

In the event of a black and white presentation, look to the coding system chosen and be guided by that. More often than not, a thin line is used for the physical cycle, a thick one for the emotional rhythm and the intellectual rhythm is shown by a dotted line. This is a good way to mark out the cycles and is a representation chosen quite some time ago.

Each card is usually made out for one calendar month with each of the cycles easily and instantly recognised. As time moved on, it meant that people could go anywhere in the world for any length of time and renew their biogram without too much of a problem. Today, however, there are some limitations in all of these ways because of a lack of the 'dedicated' calculators that are no longer available.

Most of the older books are more or less out of print and, save for a very small handful of new works that have come on the market within in the last ten years or so, what is available is workable, but has 'explanations' for the day that do vary slightly from author to author. However, the end result is almost always correct but do check everything you work out very carefully because any mistake made at this stage is most unhelpful.

What few companies who do advertise a biorhythm charting service may be counted on one hand here in the UK. However, the advent of the personal computer has created a whole range of different biorhythm programs that present your personal readings on the screen – or you may print them out as a hard-copy. While they are readily available at the touch of a button or two, they are also, for the most part, all quite reliable.

The write-up for the individual daily cycle may be a tad questionable in some cases. Whatever, they can appear on-screen as a part of the loading/switch-on program or may reside in a directory as you see fit. The hard copy print-out also varies with different programs.

For personal research purposes, I currently hold some fifteen different programs in a special directory on one of my (very) old machines along with several of the old fashioned calculators as well. In addition, I also have a variety of programs for some of the small hand-held personal computers and on top of all this, I also have a small collection of pre-printed cards along with a couple of cardboard 'wheel' calculators that came on the market with the occasional time-to-time offers that came from magazines or other sources.

Many of these programs and all of the calculator systems are or were limited to the twentieth century, starting at January 01 1901 through to December 31 1999. This makes life rather difficult for students who wish to trace the lives of historical figures.

ESTABLISHING THE BIRTH DATE

With or without a calculator, it is possible to check the biorhythms for anyone whose birth date is known. It only takes a few short minutes. This system may be confidently used for any date from September 02 1752, when Great Britain changed from the Julian calendar, having decided to adopt the new and modernised Gregorian calendar in its place.

At that time, Britain used the Julian calendar and was some eleven days adrift of other countries that had already made the change. When we changed over on Wednesday 2 September 1752, the day was followed by Thursday 14 September 1752. It should go without saying that uproar followed this with many demanding to know where their 'lost' week was and whether or not they were going to be compensated accordingly. And, of course, that year was only 355 days long.

Any date prior to this may be suspect and you should make a point of verifying your information before this particular period. The American Colonies changed at the same day and date for they were still subject to British law. However, many other countries changed at different times both before and after us.

Generally speaking, most dates referred to in books and other publications have already been converted to the new system but this is not set in tablets of stone. Almost all of the computer systems now available have had the adjustment worked out but it never hurts to double-check – just in case you have cause to make the check. Remember, some works may quote their information within the context of the calendar prevailing at the time in question but a visit to the local library ought to furnish you with the correct details.

Students of history and the then prominent historical figures who find it fascinating to delve into the pasts of heroes or villains may now add the biorhythmic aspect to their investigations. Could their biorhythms have had a bearing on the way they acted or thought at the time?

A good biography often lists the full dates of an event so, armed with this and the birthdate of the individual concerned, an hour or two may be very pleasurably and profitably passed looking to see 'the how and the why' this man or that woman possibly acted as they did. Indeed, you might also care to examine the compatibility factor between individuals or groups of people, for it might well throw further sidelights on to their relationships.

A few minutes work will give you similar results in respect of your modern favourites too, whether they are pop stars, actors or sportsmen and women. And it can be fun to work out why newscasters or other presenters may fluff their lines several times while you watch. Well-known personalities may act in a way not normally associated with them.

Golfers or other sportsmen and women may appear to be completely off-form during a particular match. A host of occasions will offer you food for thought and provide the impetus necessary to check the biorhythms of your favourite personality.

FIRST STEPS

First of all you have to learn how to work out the stages and phases of the biorhythms of the individual people concerned. To establish these points, one must determine the number of days that have elapsed from the date of birth up to the date you are interested in and here it must be stressed that you have to include the date of birth as well as the date in question in your investigation.

This total is then divided by the number of day's duration of each cycle. Thus for the physical cycle one must divide by 23. For the emotional cycle divide by 28 and for the intellectual rhythm divide by 33. In each case, the remainder figure indicates the stage of that particular rhythm. Where there is no remainder, this means that the day is a critical one and the following day will be day one of the new positive phase.

In the physical rhythm, the positive phase starts on day one and lasts until day twelve which is a critical day. The days from two through to eleven are the plus stage which peaks at a mini-critical point on day seven. From day thirteen to twenty-three is the negative stage, with the mini-critical on day eighteen.

In the emotional cycle, day one starts the positive phase, which lasts until day fifteen, the critical day. The mini-critical point is on day eight. Days two to fourteen mark the plus phase of this rhythm. The negative stage runs from day sixteen until day twenty-eight with the mini-critical occurring on day twenty-two. The intellectual rhythm starts on day one and is positive until day seventeen, which is the critical day. The mini-critical day in the cycle occurs on day nine. The negative stage lasts from day eighteen until day thirty-three, with the mini-critical taking place on the 26th.

DETERMINING BIORHYTHMS

The tables in this section have been created for you to calculate biorhythms without a calculator. For our example, we will take someone born on May 24 1950 and calculate their biorhythms for October 27 1979.

Fig 1 will help you start to find your total number of days quickly. Where the specific number of years required is not listed, combine the necessary figure to obtain the desired total.

RHYTHMS OF LIFE

1 × 365 = 365	10 × 365 = 3650
2 × 365 = 730	20 × 365 = 7300
3 × 365 = 1095	30 × 365 = 10950
4 × 365 = 1460	40 × 365 = 14600
5 × 365 = 1825	50 × 365 = 18250
6 × 365 = 2190	60 × 365 = 21900
7 × 365 = 2555	70 × 365 = 25550
8 × 365 = 2920	80 × 365 = 29200
9 × 365 = 3285	90 × 365 = 32850

Fig 1

1756	1760	1764	1768	1772	1776	1780	1784	1788
1792	1796	1804	1808	1812	1816	1820	1824	1828
1832	1836	1840	1844	1848	1852	1856	1860	1864
1868	1872	1876	1880	1884	1888	1892	1896	1900
1908	1912	1916	1920	1924	1928	1932	1936	1940
1944	1948	1952	1956	1960	1964	1968	1972	1976
1980	1984	1988	1992	1996	2004	2008	2012	2016
2020	2024	2028	2032	2036	2040	2044	2048	2052

Missing 1904.....???????

Fig 2 *Leap Years Since 1752.*

CALCULATIONS

Day	Jan	Feb	Mar	Apr	May	Jun	Jul	Aug	Sep	Oct	Nov	Dec
1	1	32	60	91	121	152	182	213	244	274	305	335
2	2	33	61	92	122	153	183	214	245	275	306	336
3	3	34	62	93	123	154	184	215	246	276	307	337
4	4	35	63	94	124	155	185	216	247	277	308	338
5	5	36	64	95	125	156	186	217	248	278	309	339
6	6	37	65	96	126	157	187	218	249	279	310	340
7	7	38	66	97	127	158	188	219	250	280	311	341
8	8	39	67	98	128	159	189	220	251	281	312	342
9	9	40	68	99	129	160	190	221	252	282	313	343
10	10	41	69	100	130	161	191	222	253	283	314	344
11	11	42	70	101	131	162	192	223	254	284	315	345
12	12	43	71	102	132	163	193	224	255	285	316	346
13	13	44	72	103	133	164	194	225	256	286	317	347
14	14	45	73	104	134	165	195	226	257	287	318	348
15	15	46	74	105	135	166	196	227	258	288	319	349
16	16	47	75	106	136	167	197	228	259	289	320	350
17	17	48	76	107	137	168	198	229	260	290	321	351
18	18	49	77	108	138	169	199	230	261	291	322	352
19	19	50	78	109	139	170	200	231	262	292	323	353
20	20	51	79	110	140	171	201	232	263	293	324	354
21	21	52	80	111	141	172	202	233	264	294	325	355
22	22	53	81	112	142	173	203	234	265	295	326	356
23	23	54	82	113	143	174	204	235	266	296	327	357
24	24	55	83	114	144	175	205	236	267	297	328	358
25	25	56	84	115	145	176	206	237	268	298	329	359
26	26	57	85	116	146	177	207	238	269	299	330	360
27	27	58	86	117	147	178	208	239	270	300	331	361
28	28	59	87	118	148	179	209	240	271	301	332	362
29	29		88	119	149	180	210	241	272	302	333	363
30	30		89	120	150	181	211	242	273	303	334	364
31	31		90		151		212	243		304		365

Fig 3 *This table has been created to show the number of each day in the year calculated progressively. In a leap year, add one (1) more day from February 28.*

On 27 October, our subject would have been 29 years old plus the extra days. Therefore, we will begin our calculations from Figure 1:

$$20 \times 365 = 7300$$
$$+ \ 9 \times 365 = 3285$$
$$\overline{10585 \text{ (days) carry forward.}}$$

From figure 2 we see the subject has lived through seven leap years, thus:

$$7$$
$$+ \ 10585$$
$$\overline{10592 \text{ (days) carry forward.}}$$

We now need to know how many days have elapsed since the birth date, 24 May 1950, until 27 October 1979. From figure 6, we see that 27 October is day 300 and that 24 May is day 144, therefore:

$$300$$
$$- \ 144$$
$$\overline{156}$$

Bring forward 10592 and add this to 156 to obtain the next figure required:

$$10592$$
$$+ \ 156$$
$$\overline{10748}$$

You must now add 1 to this figure for the day in question, thus:

$$1$$
$$+ \ 10748$$
$$\overline{10749}$$

Our subject has, therefore, lived a total of 10749 days, inclusive of the day for which we wish to calculate the biorhythms. To

> ascertain the physical rhythm we now divide this by 23. The whole figure represents the number of full cycles experienced; the remainder figure indicates the stage of the current cycle. Multiply remainders (always a decimal number) by 23 or 28 or 33 as the case may be.
> Thus:
>
> $$467 \text{ remainder } 8$$
> $$23 : 10749$$
>
> Therefore, on 27 October the physical rhythm is 8 days into the plus stage.
>
> Similarly, for the emotional rhythm we now divide 10749 by 28. Thus:
>
> $$383 \text{ remainder } 25$$
> $$28 : 10749$$
>
> On 27 October the emotional rhythm has reached day 25 of its cycle and is in the negative stage. Again, for the intellectual cycle we divide 10749 by 33. Thus:
>
> $$325 \text{ remainder } 24$$
> $$33 : 10749$$
>
> Therefore, on 27 October the intellectual rhythm is at day 24, and in the negative phase.

Fig 4

So, for our friend who was born on May 24 1950, the full biorhythmic reading for the day is 8 for the physical cycle, 25 for the sensitivity cycle and 24 for the intellectual rhythm.

The interpretation for these readings taken together might read back as '...an ideal day in which to clear up an outstanding matter, would need a little physical effort but not a lot of concentration. Turn your mind to problems that need not be resolved straight away so you could do something along the lines of taking the dog for a walk perhaps...'

DETERMINING BIORHYTHMS USING A CALCULATOR

This will certainly eliminate mathematical error and exertion. Take an ordinary calculator and work out the number of days elapsed from the date of birth to the date in question using the previous examples as before. You must remember to add one day to the total figure to account for the day under review.

Provided you used the same example as you did earlier, your total will be 10749.

Using your calculator, divide this number by 23, 28 and 33. Thus:

10749/23 = 467.34782 (physical cycle)
10749/28 = 383.89285 (emotional cycle)
10749/33 = 325.72727 (intellectual cycle)

To arrive at the physical biorhythm stage, multiply the decimal remainder by 23, thus:

.34782 × 23 = 7.99986
(to the nearest whole number, this is 8).

To establish the state of the emotional cycle, multiply the decimal remainder by 28, thus:

.89285 × 28 = 24.9998
(to the nearest whole number, this is 25).

To work out the right day for the intellectual biorhythm stage, multiply the decimal remainder by 33, thus:

.72727 × 33 = 23.99991
(to the nearest whole number, this is 24).

CALCULATIONS

Once you have worked out what the individual cycles are for any particular day, event or person, it becomes a fairly simple exercise to create a biogram for a month, or for as long as you like. You might wish to travel back in time to see why the individual person in question was average, better than average or impaired in some way. Alternatively, you may want to make up a card for a month in advance. Either way, these two examples will provide you with the best method of making basic biorhythm charts without the aid of a dedicated biorhythm calculator.

All the information you need to calculate and then put into practice what you have learned has been provided in these pages and we have also supplied a number of blank charts at the back of the book with which you may experiment (see page 000).

To carry out this task (which will get easier every time you do it), you will need four coloured pens or pencils. That will be black for the identity data, red for the physical rhythm, blue for the emotional cycle and green for the intellectual rhythm and a protractor which you will want to help you create the curves in an even fashion. This can be bought just about anywhere in most local high streets for a few pence.

When creating a biogram, try to work your calculations in such a way so that you start your biogram for the first day of the required month. It then becomes a lot easier to pick out the critical days. Draw in the curves between the points (dates) and once you have completed your first card, the next becomes easier; the next even easier until, suddenly, it is all old hat.

However, a word of caution – do check all your calculations very carefully to ensure that you have got everything right, especially for the very first time. After this, a little practice will not take long for it all to fall into place.

It is also appreciated that this might all look a tad daunting so try your hand at working out the biorhythms for just one day at first. It will make creating a card for a short period much easier especially if you are creating a card for yourself.

Here is another example to help you get into the swing of things but this time the working has been approached from a slightly different angle. We will assume we want the biorhythms for December 31 1999 for someone born June 24 1939. On December 31 1999 our subject would be sixty years old.

Thus, the whole calculation is: 60×365 + leap year days + days from 24 June + 1.

From figure 1, we get $60 \times 365 = 21900$.
From figure 2, the leap years from 1939 until 1999 equal 15.
Thus:

$$\begin{array}{r} 21900 \\ +15 \\ \hline 21915 \end{array}$$

From figure 3, we find that December 31 is equal to 365 days and that June 24 is the 175th day.
Thus:

$$\begin{array}{r} 365 \\ -175 \\ \hline 190 \end{array}$$

Thus:

$$\begin{array}{r} 190 \\ +\,21915 \\ \hline 22105 \end{array}$$

$$\begin{array}{r} +\,1 \\ \hline 22106 \end{array} \text{(for the day in question)}$$

We now divide this total figure by the relative cycle lengths: 23 for the physical rhythm, 28 for the emotional rhythm and 33 for the intellectual rhythm.

CALCULATIONS

We will do this first without a calculator.

Physical: 961 remainder 3
               23 :22106

Emotional: 789 remainder 14
               28 :22106

Intellectual: 669 remainder 29
               33 :22106

The biorhythms for this individual on December 31 1999 work out as follows: The physical rhythm is at day 3, the emotional cycle is at day 14 (a critical day) and the intellectual cycle is at day 29.

When we use the calculator method we will also use the figure of 22106 for that is the total number of days that have elapsed from the date of birth until the day in question. We then divide this number by the amount of days of each cycle.

Thus:

$$22106/23 = 961.13043 \text{ (physical cycle)}$$
$$22106/28 = 789.5 \quad \text{(emotional cycle)}$$
$$22106/23 = 669.87878 \text{ (intellectual cycle)}$$

To arrive at the day the of cycle length involved we multiply the remainder by the length of days in that cycle.

Thus:

For the physical cycle multiply by 23:
.3043 × 23 = 2.99989 (which to the nearest whole number is 3)

For the emotional cycle multiply by 28:
.5 × 28 = 14 (straightforward result and a critical day)

For the intellectual cycle multiply by 33:
.87878 × 33 = 28.99974 (which to the nearest whole number is 29)

The biorhythms on December 31 1999 for someone born on June 24 1939 therefore are for the physical cycle, day 3; the emotional cycle, day 14; and intellectual cycle, day 29.

Biorhythmically, this might be read as '…Feeling fairly good physically but emotionally this individual could be a little restless.' Their overall judgment, however, might be suspect and it would be a good idea to allow the day go by and just rely on what sixth sense he or she may have. By deferring important decisions today they ought not to be tempted into making mistakes.

After you have carried out a few of these exercises yourself, it will soon be relatively easy and much quicker to determine these calculations. You should practice with friends and relatives or anyone else with whom you can speak and who either attracts your interest or actually asks you to do the work.

In the appendix of this book are the birthdates of quite a few well known people from all walks of life: history, sport, politics and the entertainment world along with a host of individuals who have made a niche for themselves in the pages of history by their actions, thoughts or words. The list also includes both the famous and the infamous.

The prime directive here is to remember that biorhythms do not in themselves have a cause and effect but are subject to the prevailing conditions of the moment. You will find that the phase of their cycles at the time of their actions you may be questioning could well have had a bearing on why these people acted as they did.

It will also come as quite a surprise to discover the basis of a famous (or infamous) partnership, biorhythmically speaking. Not everyone needs to be of the same thinking or emotional, although in some cases this doesn't always hurt. There are times when one partner may do better to be in a position to lead the other one in certain circumstances.

However, this should not always concern you for you are there to learn and report. You can always go through a past event with a client or the people concerned in your investigation. On many an occasion, you will find that it may be patently obvious why this happened or that did not take place at times.

However, in respect of what one might suggest that people should do in respect of something that is to take place at a later date is quite different.

And that is what this work is all about, learning how to apply the theory of cyclic behaviour patterns through biorhythmic cycles. With a little judicial application, you can soon learn how live with your biorhythms, and those of other folk in order to experience a more satisfactory way of life – in every sense of the word.

CHAPTER 7

THE DAILY BIORHYTHM

Every day and in one way or another, we all experience one of 27 different basic phases or stages in our biorhythms. These combinations have been very carefully studied for a long time and the daily readings as set out below are a fair assessment of what to expect.

However, it would be wiser to use them as a guide only for none of them should be regarded as being set in tablets of stone.

Please remember that these ideas are suggestions only as to what you might be reasonably expected to experience.

For each of the critical days, no allowance has been made for the direction of the phase – only that it is a critical day.

There are 27 possible variations in the whole of the one day biorhythm scene.

H = Positive Phase
X = Critical Day
L = Negative Stage

LLL
When all three rhythms are marked at their lowest point, you will be well under your normal strengths all round. It would better to just let things happen as they will. It would be safer to start nothing new, no matter how strongly you might feel. Mistakes could prove to be quite costly.

HLL
Physically, you should be able to tackle most things but let others take the lead when it comes to thinking through the strategy for the day. Think twice and check before you commit yourself to anything. Whatever attracts you emotionally will only be a passing moment or two and not last for long.

HHL
It might be better to allow your sixth sense to work for you today. You will feel in fine fettle and well able to undertake most outstanding tasks. However, no matter how you feel something will go well, your judgment cannot be relied upon but for the most part this should be a good day.

HHH
Such a time does not come around that often but when it does. make the most of it, for everything should go your way. With all three cycles in their positive states, it means this is your time. Make sure you have the right people around to help you maximise on all you want to do.

LHH
The mind and heart are more than willing but you probably feel that you simply don't have the energy to try getting anything done. It will be a trying and tiring time if you do try to keep up with everything and everybody. It would be better to plan for what is really important.

LLH
You will be far better off on your own mainly because your temper might easily become frayed at the edges. People may seem annoying but it isn't them – it is you. You know what you want but you could be unable to attain your ambitions today. Avoid social gatherings if you can.

LHL
You won't feel as if you are in among the leadership stakes today but you will almost certainly be quite confident about some of your ideas for implementing later. Energy levels are rather low at this time. Might be better to spend time with your hobbies or pastimes or people who you trust.

HLH
Physically you are in fine fettle and your mind may be working overtime but emotionally you are at a low ebb and even a tad depressed. Your social life won't go that well if you attempt to be a leader. It might be better to keep a low profile and play the lone wolf.

LLX
This is an incident and or an accident prone period. Don't be tempted to take risks or you will be the loser. You will probably feel low on all three levels but this is an intellectual critical day. You will be unable to think straight so don't be tempted into doing anything out of the ordinary.

LHX
This is another one of those incident or accident prone days. Emotionally, you and that very special person should get along quite well together. New people in your circle will be welcomed. However, physically you will feel a tad out of it and on an intellectual critical day trouble could be looming.

HLX
One shouldn't be put off by the term 'intellectual critical day' for it implies is that your thinking will be flawed in some way. Having your physical energies liable to be dissipated in some way and your emotional responses to be a tad over the top suggests another incident and accident prone day.

HHX
Today you should be ultra-careful, for your physical high combined with an emotional high implies a level of self-delusion you can ill afford, especially as your thinking isn't straight and, as serious errors of judgment are likely, it might lead you into a potentially incident and accident prone day.

LXL
With an intellectual low, physically negative and emotionally critical short period like this it really isn't your day at all. You would be much better off delegating where you can or, if you cannot do so then by all means go ahead but any effort you do make should be made with great caution.

LXH
There will be a tendency to be over confident thinking about anything new because you can't pursue things with your normal vim and vigour. On an emotional critical day you are rather prone to be irritable because you can't take criticism, no matter how well meant. This is an incident and accident prone period.

HXL
Physically you are at the peak of your powers but may end up at odds with everyone else because you are liable to fail to grasp important points that anyone else will easily spot. You won't be that sociable either because of the emotional critical time. Be careful if revising or writing up notes.

HXH
Not the best of times for driving yourself anywhere because you are likely to be a tad over confident but there will be a lack of concentration and this makes you incident or accident prone. You may also be a trifle irritable with either yourself or those around you who might criticise.

XLL

This rather short serious accident prone period is one where, if anything is to go wrong, it will be around now. You must be very careful at all times not only for your own safety but also for those around you. You will lack foresight and should keep a low profile.

XLH

Once again, this implies the possibility of incidents and accidents that can be avoided if you heed the advice of those around you. You will feel physically tired, low emotionally and unlikely to suffer fools. Keep an open mind, for any distractions could cost and not necessarily just in terms of cash.

XHH

Emotionally and intellectually you will be at your best, but don't try to over-do it, from a physical standpoint. It is nice to think that you are not vulnerable but you can't do whatever you want. This is another incident and accident prone period. Be careful in what you say or do.

XHL

A fundamentally low period because you will be more than just a tad uncoordinated in all you try to do today. You are far too eager to please or will want be seen in a better light than you actually feel. Mishaps, mistakes and errors are much more likely unless you slow down.

LXX

Both your emotional and intellectual rhythms are in a critical phase today. You may well feel off-balance or unable to keep up with what is going on. A low phase physical cycle really doesn't help at all here and is liable to make things worse. Try to avoid physical activities that need good coordination.

HXX
Both your emotional and intellectual ability could be stretched to the limit. Your physical levels are at a high point and sport of some kind would be welcome, even it is only a morning jog. You may feel fine but this a risky day for starting anything new.

XLX
Rather wearing all round with people seemingly uncooperative or just plain awkward. This will probably be you and your perception of things because of your low emotional state that won't help your temper either. You are accident prone, in that you may assess people and or things wrongly and for all the wrong reasons.

XHX
Keep your eyes open, for you are likely to not see the warning signs because you feel so good. As both your physical and intellectual cycles are in critical phases, the chances are you could make many mistakes today. Blaming others for your errors won't help your cause at all.

XXH
When your rhythms are physically and emotionally critical there is always a danger of serious mistakes occurring when you least expect them. Driving is not recommended and nor is too much travel of any kind. This could be quite an awkward short period, so do take the time to think things through.

XXL
Another short period in which you shouldn't drive and, in fact, taken all round, it might be best if you kept a low profile and just handled only what was absolutely necessary. You won't be able to see the wood for trees and if you can, you should accept this as another accident prone period.

XXX
A day like this rarely occurs. Sit tight, do nothing and stay cool, calm and collected for as long as you can. Take the day off and spend time with your hobbies unless they need concentration, in which case forgo this pleasure as well. Start nothing and, preferably, try not to finish anything either.

THE PHYSICAL CYCLE

The first phase of this rhythm permits full participation in almost any kind of physical activity without worry. You feel good and on top of the world, nothing is too much of an effort.

When in the second phase, try to ease back. You may feel less enthusiasm for anything physical. It can be difficult to keep up. On a critical day, try to avoid unnecessary exercise or activity, you could be accident-prone.

THE SENSITIVITY CYCLE

This rhythm is concerned mainly with your mood and social ability. In the first part of the cycle you are cheerful, co-operative and more optimistic. You will shine socially and are inclined to be more creative in your overall outlook.

In the second or negative stage you may be moody, touchy and uncooperative. You become tense and liable to be irritable and feel low. On a critical day, you are ultra-sensitive and easily stressed. Accidents are known to take place as a result.

THE INTELLECTUAL CYCLE

In the first or plus stage, your logic and reasoning powers are at their best. You are perceptive and your ideas and responses flow fluidly. Problems are easily resolved, concentration is easy and you should use the time for study periods.

In the second or negative stage, your perception rate and understanding levels tend to drop quite noticeably and your memory is likely to be faulty. On a critical day, intelligence is muddled, silly mistakes are made and accidents happen through poor judgement.

HOW TO READ A BIO-CHART

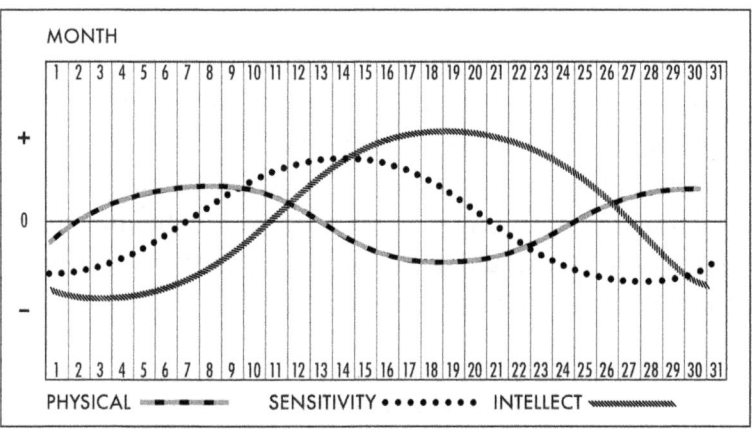

In the illustration, the first critical day is in the physical cycle where it changes from the negative stage to the positive stage on the 2nd day. It then passes from positive to negative on the 13th and returns to the first phase again on the 25th where it ends the month. The emotional cycle has its first critical day passing from the negative stage to the plus on the 7th. It returns to the negative phase again on the 21st where it ends the month. The intellectual cycle is in critical phase as it passes from the negative to the positive on the 11th. It returns to the negative stage on the 27th where it ends the month.

PRACTICAL BIORHYTHMS

When we have our bio-charts to consult, we are far better able to time our performances. It is always to our advantage when we are at our best – biorhythmically speaking, of course.

Whole new worlds of experience open up. We know now how to time matters to our benefit and not just because it is the next job on the list. We know now how to arrange things so that we have all that extra energy to use much more constructively than before. We may also have enough energy left over to pour into other daily events and any unnecessary tiredness can become a thing of the past.

Look at the bio-chart again. There is little point in digging over the garden between the 13th and 25th unless it is absolutely necessary because it is a backbreaking task, to say the least. By waiting until you are in the positive stage, you would be able to tackle the job in half the time, twice as effectively and with half the effort.

There is nothing to stop you tackling the task between these dates, just take it easy and conserve your strength to avoid over doing it.

According to the chart, the emotional rhythm suggests the best time to attend or give a party would be between the 8th and the 20th because you will be in fine fettle throughout. If you really want to shine and be at your best, select a day at least five or six days after a negative to positive critical day. It would be helpful if the other two cycles could be favourable but if they are not then simply make the necessary compensations to allow for the individual phases on the day.

If you can name the date for an important business event, you should always elect for a positive intellectual day. Your mind will be crisp, alert and sufficiently perceptive to deal with all the expected and the unexpected problems that can happen at such times. According to this chart, the best dates would be between the 13th and the 25th.

Obviously, where a task or an activity has to be dealt with when in an unfavourable stage of a cycle, stop, think and elect to adapt, conserve and adjust what available energies you do have to best suit your cause.

Learn to use your biorhythms to the best advantage – yours!

CHAPTER 8

COMPATIBILITY

We all need to get along as best we can with the people with whom we work, friends, neighbours and to a greater or lesser extent our family relations, whether they may have been 'inherited' by marriage or those with whom we grew up.

So often this compatibility can be quite uncertain. We might behave almost irrationally towards someone we meet for the first time when something does not seem to quite 'click' into place. In effect, whatever bond we might have expected just doesn't materialise at all. Even worse, as time wears on, something that you may feel about this new acquaintanceship just fails to get off the ground altogether.

However, on another occasion we seem to achieve an ideal rapport because we appear to have so much common ground where we are able to think along similar lines and can enjoy each other's company more or less all the time.

If we were to now compare our biorhythm charts, the solution might be easily found. We may be able to pinpoint an apparent discrepancy or find a favourable outlook in this new relationship. After all, it is a logical step to propose that what biorhythms 'do' for you, they must 'do' for others.

While reactions to personal biorhythms can and do vary from individual to individual, they can so often provide guidelines as to how we ought to relate successfully with other folk. Just as easily, they will also be able to help us find out where we need to build bridges to maintain the new associations.

BIORHYTHMIC COMPATIBILITY

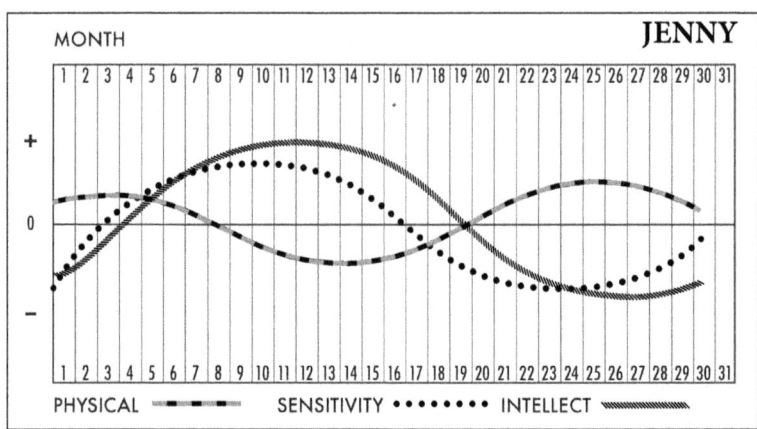

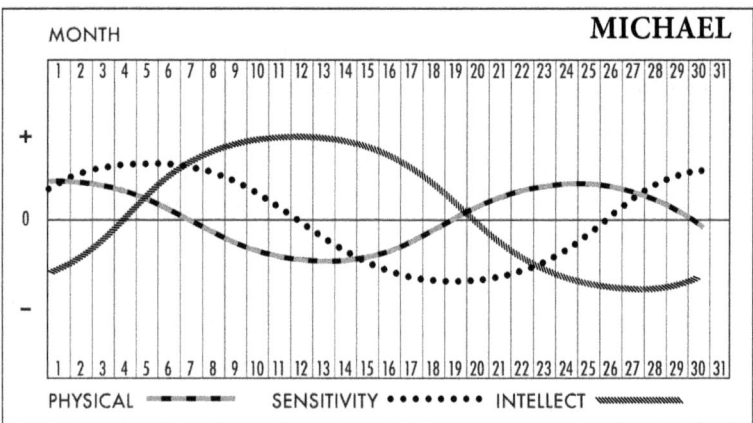

When you look at the first two illustrations you will see quite a bit of similarity between them. In this case, both individuals experience intellectual critical days on the 4th and 20th. Jenny (the subject of the first chart) has her first physical critical day on the 8th and then another one on the 20th. Michael, the second subject, experiences his physical critical days on the 7th and 19th. Their emotional critical periods differ much more widely. Hers are on the 3rd and 17th while his are on the 12th and 26th of the month.

COMPATIBILITY

So, in this study of compatibility, Jenny and Michael share the same phases of their intellectual cycles, are one day apart in the their physical rhythms but are nine days adrift in their emotional rhythms. We can see immediately that these two young people more or less think and act alike, have an almost imperceptible difference in their physical lives but are fairly different when it comes to an appraisal of their emotional approach to life. When they first met, they got on well from day one and have been relatively good friends since.

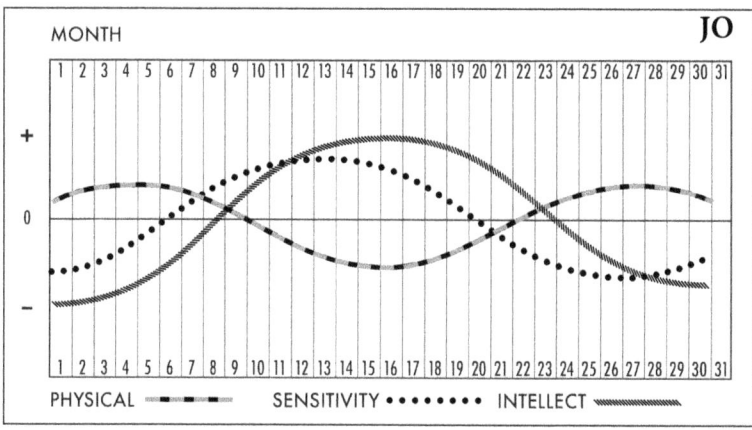

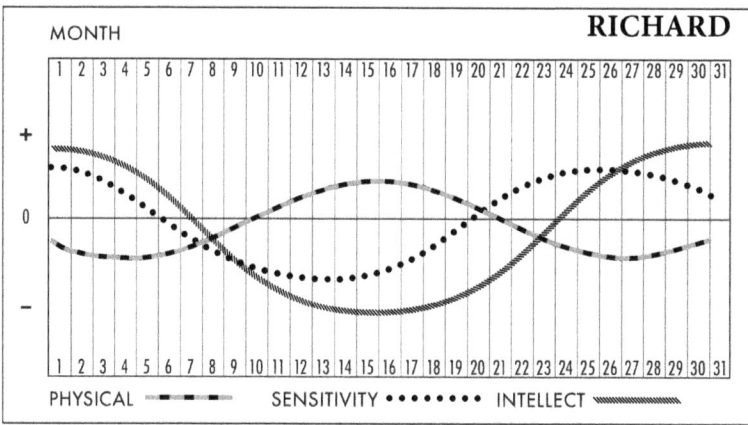

The two people we chose for this study, Jo and Richard, are of a quite different pairing altogether. You will see that they both experience emotional critical days on the same day, but their cycles are in opposing phases. Jenny's emotional positive stage runs from the 6th through until the 20th while Richard experiences his in reverse. He enters his emotional negative stage on the 6th but returns to his positive phase in this cycle on the 20th.

Jo has her first physical critical day 10th and moves back into the positive phase again on the 22nd. Richard, however, is the reverse of this in that his first physical critical day from negative to positive is on the 10th and returns to the negative phase on the 21st. Their Intellectual biorhythms are one day apart. Jo has her first intellectual critical day on the 8th when she enters her positive phase and returns to her negative stage on the 24th. Richard has his on the 7th day when he enters his negative stage of this cycle on the 7th but changes back to the positive phase on the 24th.

COMPATIBILITY RATINGS

When we assess the compatibility rating of these two pairs we find that Jenny and Michael have an overall rating of 85% which is fairly high. These ratings are created from a 91% physical compatibility, 64% emotional and 100% in their intellectual compatibility.

Jo and Richard have much less than this. Their overall figure is a mere 7% made up from 4% in their physical cycles, 0% in the emotional rhythm and only 3% intellectually. These are, of course, very low figures indeed.

Both pairs are taken from life. These four people get along with each other as best as they can. Jenny and Michael are (very) good friends while Jo and Richard just work with each other. Even before I assessed the relationships of both couples, Jenny and Michael seemed to appreciate they did get on well but Jo and Richard knew in their heart of hearts that they had to work hard to maintain some semblance of order between them.

Once I had explained these differences, they get along far better, although their personalities still remain much the same. In simple terms, they realised that they had to get along with each other for business purposes. They thought a lot more about it and eventually, made a few changes here and there and now get along a little better than before but at least they now understand why.

To assess compatibility, you calculate the difference between the individual's cycles in days, for each one represents a proportion of the problem or problems a couple, or more than just two people in some cases, are likely to encounter.

Add the difference in days for each cycle to obtain the overall figure. Divide the total by three because there are only three cycles (at present) that are assessed. The result is the total compatibility rating and it remains constant throughout the life. Later, we will move on to look at cycles other than these three principal rhythms when we assess compatibility. In such cases, we note the number of cycles used and divide by that amount.

Some biorhythm exponents feel that this total ought to be read only as a guide, while others feel that this is the right way to compare character and personality differences. On top of that, it has been noticed that the rhythm that reports the highest percentage figure in the overall total does reflect most strongly in the relationship.

So, if you recall, the figures we arrived at with Jenny and Michael were 91%, 64% and 100% making the main point of interest between them in the intellectual cycle. Their association is well noted by others around them because they all agree that they seem to possess an almost uncanny ability to read each other's minds at times. Not only do they both have a similar approach to life, they also seem to have rather similar emotional ideals as well.

Where Jo and Richard are concerned, their very low total reflects their ability to get on. These figures were 4% for their physical rhythms, 0% for their emotional cycles and just 3% for their intellectual rhythms. These totals are so small and close they really do have nothing in common at all. Unfortunately, there is no key factor from which we could try to work – they just have nothing in common.

PHYSICAL COMPATIBILITY

The higher the compatibility factor in the physical rhythm, the more readily you are prepared to take part in work or games that need an equal amount of effort by both (or more) people. Sport especially usually relies on this kind of combined equal effort if the undertaking is to be properly enjoyed.

For example, if you were to ask two people to climb a steep cliff, they would each have to rely on the other to pull their weight. If this is not possible, one must assume leadership while the other should step back to allow this. Otherwise it isn't going to be a very pleasant time for either of them.

EMOTIONAL COMPATIBILITY

When we come to evaluate the biorhythmic emotional compatibility between subjects, the maximum rating is quite acceptable for most relationships except, perhaps, for long term associations such as marriage, simply living together and or certain family associations. The closer the subject couple (or more) may be the more they are going to share the same kind of response to whatever may beset them at the time for good or ill. Similar rhythms will lead to tension, for by experiencing the same 'highs' and 'lows' and the same critical days, will not only prove to be boring but it might cause as many problems as incompatible folk may share.

If there is insufficient emotional stimulation, the association may well fail on a temporary basis perhaps, but if the partners are in a bad mood on a negative critical day, heaven help them and those around them. The best rating for married people is around 45% – 65% because there will be a consistent stimulus as their cycles are always slightly out of step. Below this rating will make the partners concerned to have to exercise tact, timing and understanding in anything where emotional rapport would be helpful.

INTELLECTUAL COMPATIBILITY

Any lack of stimulation here may be due to a poor compatibility rating, so when we arrive at a 100% in our assessment it will provide excellent results in most relationships but there might be a few odd problems here and there because the subjects will have 'think-alike' ideas. The best figure here would be about 75% because the one can lead and complement the other, should their cycles vary that much. Partner No. 1 will be able to guide and lead partner No. 2 when he or she is in an obviously better condition. These roles can change when it becomes time for the other one to hold the reins. Generally speaking, the assessment of around 50% or slightly lower will prove to be about the best.

Although there will obviously be a contrasting intellectual approach requiring a certain amount of tact, once the reason has been explained, those involved can apply themselves a lot more diligently than in previous times. Partners will soon learn to allow for the differences in their perception rates and time their best moments for those all-important joint decisions.

The higher the overall compatibility rating, the better the relationship should be but it almost certainly will be coloured

COMPATIBILITY TABLE

DAYS APART IN CYCLE	PHYSICAL CYCLE %	EMOTIONAL CYCLE %	INTELLECTUAL CYCLE %
0	100	100	100
1	91	93	94
2	83	86	88
3	74	79	82
4	65	71	76
5	57	64	70
6	48	57	64
7	39	50	58
8	30	43	52
9	22	36	46
10	13	29	39
11	4	21	33
12	4	14	27
13	13	7	21
14	22	0	15
15	30	7	9
16	39	14	3
17	48	21	3
18	57	29	9
19	65	36	15
20	74	43	21
21	83	50	27
22	91	57	33
23	100	64	39
24		71	46
25		79	52
26		86	58
27		93	64
28		100	70
29			76
30			82
31			88
32			94
33			100

COMPATIBILITY

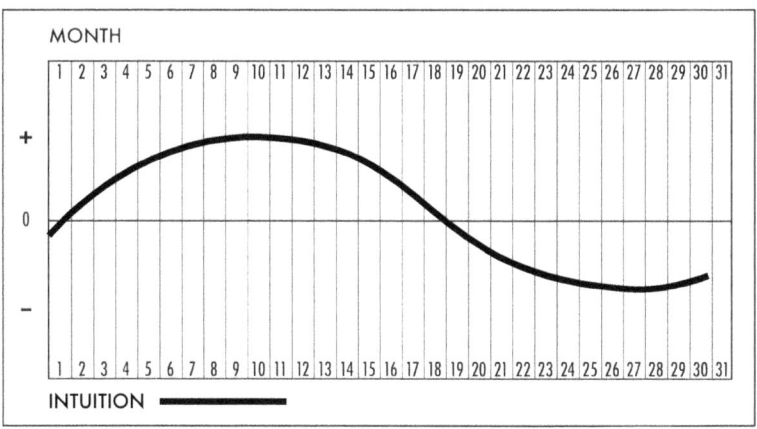

by the cycle with the highest percentage. So, when the physical rating is the highest, the relationship will rely on their ability to enjoy each other's physical presence. When the highest figure is in the emotional cycle, they are temperamentally suited; and should it be that the intellectual relationship is accentuated, then they are mentally attuned.

Add the results together and divide by three to arrive at the overall compatibility figure.

GROUP COMPATIBILITY

Any amount of subjects may be used to assess compatibility. We can rate as many people as necessary to ensure the arena of activity with which they are involved or for an event that may be in the planning mode for a later date. We are able to improve and make better working conditions and relationships at the same time. When this work is carried out, it is done so to allow all concerned to maximise their potential at all times. Such thinking has to be along the lines of everyone to be more positive, which has to lead to better results all round.

For example, the problems that confront the modern day football team manager when selecting the best players from his list for the Saturday match suggests that an intelligent use of biorhythms will go a long way to help him maximise the potential of his best players for the day in question.

As a rule, he might normally select his team from those who seem to be at the peak of their performance. Biorhythm charts would obviously help here but might not necessarily serve to achieve the best result. Of course, a certain amount of non-compatibility will be extant in any sporting group for a variety of reasons. Most clubs have so many players at their beck and call and it is just as well for they have to take into account substitutes, reserve team players and trainees.

Thus, step one would be for these individuals to get along with each other on and off the field. The biorhythm exponent must assess the compatibility between players, the manager and each other. Once this has been worked out, the next step is to select as many of the 'star' players as far as possible but they might not all get along with each other.

With this in mind, the selection of the best possible team from a biorhythmic standpoint then becomes an easy task. However, it might still not work out too well because it could be wrong to select players at the peak of their biorhythmic positive stages, for there would be less of a 'team' performance. Each player would probably feel that he was fully capable of winning by his efforts alone. Any selection should reflect the best of the positive physical stage for each man with and also where is the most appropriate.

Unless a marked degree of emotional incompatibility exists in here anywhere, the team's emotional phasing need not necessarily be high. However, what is wanted is a high degree of Intellectual rapport because of the need for concentration. Even if the players were at their peak in their cycles, they could easily lose the game because of an inability to perform well as a team.

In spite of the fact that it is a quite dissimilar sport, cricket does call for a totally different set of skills which, in turn, requires a rather fresh approach when it comes to assessing what is needed for a successful side. The batting section of the team must have a steady eye which calls for the intellectual phase to be in its positive phase. It would also help if their physical rhythm was in the physical plus stage as well. Because a bowler has to be properly attuned his emotional rhythm should be positive and it would help for him to deliver balls accurately, consistently and powerfully. His physical rhythm, therefore, should be in the positive stage.

The tennis player always has to have reserves of energy and stamina as well as good concentration. It is asking a bit much but all of his or her biorhythms should be positive. If one claims that the serve has to be accurate and successful then this is especially so. Although we appreciate that the physical and emotional cycles should be positive, the intellectual rhythm really does have to be equally so for the player to make accurate decisions.

As with all professional sports, once the basics are mastered then the actual play tends to become second nature. Generally speaking, the accent is placed on his or her intellectual state, followed by their emotional and physical rhythms, to be sufficiently supportive for success.

A close friend sympathetic to the principles of biorhythms, especially compatibility, asked me to assess what might be wrong with a particular section of a fairly busy department store where he worked. In such a place, people have to get along with each other and their customers in some rather awkward conditions, most of the time. My immediate thoughts were that the staff could only benefit from being aware of their personal rhythms and the necessary compatibility such conditions needed.

Apart from alternate selling techniques, which differed greatly from person to person, there was also a certain amount of friction within the group. It was immediately obvious that the main cause of this stemmed from an unsuitable manager

A						
15	B					
64	91	C				
47	85	79	D			
70	86	89	92	E		
30	100	94	86	80	F	
10	18	24	12	15	33	G

A = Department Manager
G = Odd Man Out

Fig 6

who really did not get along at all well with all of his staff as well as he could have done.

In fig 6, 'A' was the departmental manager and, as you can see, he got along fairly well with two of his staff but not so well with the rest. Higher management agreed to try to resolve the matter by transferring the manager to another section to head up a different sales team where it was hoped that, once there, he would be more compatible with the staff in that section. A new head of sales was offered to the original department, which soon resulted in a happier group with a much improved sales performance all round.

One other improvement that could have been made was to have put 'G', the odd man out in this original group, into another section. If they had done so, it may have proved mutually beneficial for all concerned, as 'G' just could not get along with anyone.

If these circumstances were transferred to a factory environment, the inherent dangers soon become apparent. Conveyor-belt production techniques are monotonous and can lead to boredom and irritation, frequently resulting in accidents. In some places, employees may have to share machinery for short periods. Incompatibility along with the need for bursts of absolute concentration can soon lead to accidents, if not closely monitored. When accident rates are raised, so are insurance costs and the tempers of management. Returning to figure 6, were 'G' to be made foreman in such an environment, the turnover of staff would probably be very high indeed.

Among library staff personnel assessed it was found that, although almost everyone did get along in their intellectual phasing, their emotional and physical assessment ratings were not good at all. This is a good example of working conditions attracting people who have the ability to do a specific type of job, but not necessarily the ability to get along with each other.

The incident rate of incompatibility was frequently quite high in the old style typing pool staffed by young girls. Supervisors used to have their work cut out with exercising discipline combined with understanding. Physical compatibility was not really that important but, emotionally and intellectually, there would always have been a need to use a variety of discretionary powers.

This was best achieved through the supervisor giving certain roles to those who showed an aptitude for that specific task. This might have led to other problems, but as long as staff were given adequate explanations, then biorhythmic compatibility assessment of the employees involved served to improve their output. Depending on how you view such matters, the proliferation of computers has taken care of this particular work.

As a rule, and only if they spot what is going on, most people will try to improve their relationships with others if explanations and guidelines are offered. You may not really understand why you have never got along with him yet have always got along with her, but most folk are willing to try and improve a poor relationship even when there may be little or no guarantee of success.

Biorhythms may reveal a potential solution to the problem, but it should be remembered that compatibility is subject to personal behavioural patterns and the prevailing conditions of the moment. While the percentage figures are constant, for the best results, personal biorhythm charts should be calculated so that mutually advantageous times for joint activities can be arranged. The overall assessment figures ought really to be regarded as a guide only. It is the individual cycle figures which are the most important.

Starting a new relationship with anyone will benefit from a check of your compatibility assessment. Don't worry too much if the intellectual cycle is high but the other two are rather low by comparison. Work on the weak points in this association and business projects will prosper. And remember, even if your ratings are poor, it does not follow that you cannot be successful. You will just have to work a little bit harder at maintaining the status quo in those areas where you are at the widest variance.

Young couples considering marriage may well be a little dismayed by a poor emotional assessment but, as has already been shown, this has proved to be an almost standard result in any long-term successful associations and or marriage.

This will also be the case in a teacher/pupil relationship, driver/conductor, doctor/nurse and a nurse and patient as well. Where a new association begins between a patient who is to be looked after by a specialist nurse; then both should have their compatibility assessed for a better mutual understanding. As improvements start to show, potential physical, emotional or intellectual problems can all be made easier through long-term planning based on biorhythmic knowledge.

Such insight into your good days and bad must help all of your relationships in the long run.

CHAPTER 9

PRACTICAL CYCLES

There are very few areas where the principles of biorhythms cannot be applied. But in order to be able to apply the theory into practice, you must learn to be adaptable. Stop to re-assess what might seem to be a doubtful possibility and you ought to be able to turn the problem into a positive advantage for you and or your client.

Business people who sit in their offices are equally as prone to making poor decisions when their biorhythms are in their negative phasing, as is the third or fourth man or woman along the conveyor belt on the factory floor. Both people are likely to create terrible trouble for those around them if they make even the slightest of mistakes.

These days, this is so much so that many companies are now taking a more positive attitude and subsequent active interest in the theory and practice of the cyclic performance of the employer, manager and worker alike. In every case that has been recorded there has been a much improved performance. This has resulted in better productivity which, in turn, has meant more prosperity for all.

BUSINESS EFFICIENCY

In these modern times, business efficiency and all that goes with it has become more and more of a priority in most organisations. With the advent of computers and the leaps and bounds of today's much improved hardware along with all their associated software techniques, which require more and more people to be familiar and more highly skilled than ever. In the last 20 to 30 years or so, computers have virtually disposed of the old familiar typing pool and that has meant that even managerial types now have to write their own letters, send emails or perform other tasks that we always used to associate with those once invaluable ladies.

So, this also now means we need to know how to time events and learn not only the best methods of travel but also when to make the right moves, at the right time and for all the right reasons. Staying in touch with everyone has been considerably easier with the proliferation of the mobile phone and, in quite recent times, the tablet computer. This has brought about the relatively new inter-company 'network' gatherings that use these computer links. These days, most of us tend to take all this in our stride as a matter of course.

We have to make speedy decisions and have plenty of energy in order for us to display extreme efficiency at managing both our time and that of the people we control. To succeed in business, therefore, depends on a very high level of personal performance all the time. There is hardly any let-up these days.

Timing is all important, so it must be helpful to have not only your own biorhythm chart created for you but also those of your clients, managers, and even (especially?) your own staff as well. Once you have them it is very easy to make the simple adjustments necessary that you may wish or have to put in place. For as long as you remember to defer major decision making on a critical day, you will soon make far fewer errors of judgment that can be quite costly.

Use the negative stages of your cycles for the ordinary day-to-day routine matters. When in the positive phase, it will be easier for you to grasp new ideas and have the wherewithal to test them. You can take long, tiring business trips without drawing too much on your reserves and, in some cases, even feel the better for it. Learn to plan business meetings around your own biorhythms, especially if they are with people with whom you want to do more business.

This is one of the new tactics used in quite a few organisations these days. Executives make the effort to invest in a potential client's biorhythm calendar for several reasons. They assess the degree of compatibility and, if these figures are not too favourable, they try to find a colleague who is and turn the case file over to him or her. Deals are won on much less at times. You see, this way you hold an advantage over your opposition that, if used diligently, must help you to come out on top.

When your physical rhythm is in its positive phase, you have the necessary energy needed to maintain the effort without too much trouble. Keep up the momentum; push yourself and those who work with you to ensure you achieve your goals. Should your physical rhythm be in the negative stage, take it easy and don't be afraid to delegate. Don't try to overdo anything, play down business lunches and similar gatherings and ensure you get adequate rest. If you overdo anything now, your body is likely to rebel and let you down at just the wrong moment. The positive emotional rhythm phase is when you have the drive to carry out the tried and trusted ways and also the best time to test out new theories. You are at your peak – capitalise on it.

In the emotional cycle, the negative phase is the best time to carry out routine matters and read through notes. Plan by all means, but not too seriously. It is a rather nice time to attend or give lectures or seminars. As the tendency is to give hand-outs at the end of such gatherings, it will also save you unnecessary concentration.

The intellectual rhythm's positive phase is best used for long-term planning or for preparing reports to be read by those who matter – the boss. In the negative phase of this cycle, stick to routine, plod away at what is necessary to keep the wheels turning. Remember, there is just a chance that your memory may fail you, so stay out of the limelight. If you follow these simple rules, your personal performance will be greatly improved. This can only lead to more responsibility and promotion.

TRAVELLING

One of the many trials and tribulations of a successful business man or woman lies with his or her travel arrangements and how they either organise things or simply accept what others may have done in their name. Many problems can be easily alleviated if being driven or if public transport is used. Whatever the stage any of your rhythms may be, the trick is to ensure your comfort and well-being are catered for properly, so always allow more than enough time for your travel. After a particularly trying journey, you can always rest up prior to whatever the business commitment may demand of you.

MOTORING

When using the company car or, indeed, any other any vehicle for that matter, it is more for the driver's personal convenience than anything else. Of course, you may have to take materials which need to be used as samples or for other purposes. While safety and costs may be rather important details, with the right planning such things should never be that much of headaches for anyone. You must look up the state of your own biorhythms before making travel plans. It doesn't take that long before you learn how and when to choose the most propitious times.

You should try to avoid journeys of any length should any of your cycles be likely to be in a critical phase, irrespective of which direction they may be heading. This is especially so when the emotional rhythm is in a critical stage, for this when you are so easily irritated, become short tempered and take more chances than normal. Waiting in traffic jams, even at the traffic lights is a bore. You are liable to miss a gear, stall the engine or not see the jay-walker you would normally observe on any other day.

On an intellectually critical day, parking can prove difficult for you may be unable to gauge gaps between other vehicles properly. On a physical critical day, poor overtaking techniques tend to be the main problem. More accidents involving speed occur with those whose physical rhythms are in critical phase than at any other.

The best time for long car journeys is with your intellectual rhythm in the negative stage but with the physical and emotional rhythms in positive stages. You will not feel tired, even after a long trip, and you will be much easier to get along with. As long as you are aware of your biorhythms and compensate accordingly, all your journeys can be peaceful and safe.

DIETARY MATTERS

It is almost always the wrong time of the day, week, month or year when we suddenly find the bathroom scales, leap on them and wonder where all the extra pounds have come from. Crash diets are so often the immediate (and wrong) answer for many. Suddenly, we avoid bread, potatoes, sticky buns, we ease off the drink and (try to) take more exercise.

The result of all this extra and quite unnecessary effort tends to be a tad dramatic. One minute we are abusing our body and over-indulging in all the wrong things, the next it is hardly being cared for at all. In fact, such behaviour patterns are liable to cause really serious problems if allowed to go too far or started at the wrong stage of the physical rhythm because it might actually create more damage than it is meant to cure.

However, with proper planning and started at the right time, you should be able to create and stay with a sensible regime to help you become trim again. First of all, create your biorhythm calendar for about three to four months or so in advance, making sure that you highlight the emotional and intellectual critical days of each cycle very clearly.

For the best results, begin your new regime some seven or eight days before the first of the critical days in either cycle are due and, if possible, in the middle of the plus phase of your physical rhythm. And please remember, it isn't a good idea to wait around for such ideal conditions to materialise or you may never start.

You have to be careful of what you eat on physical critical days, so try to ensure that you eat only special diet style meals. Ignore the high starch foods like bread, potatoes, doughnuts and cream buns. However, if you feel you can't do without some sort of a nibble then prepare a few lettuce leaves, a raw carrot or a stick of celery or two. Only on this one day should it be really necessary.

As each of the critical days come along, you might find it hard initially. Strengthen your resolve during the first few critical days because, after that, it gets easier. Monitoring what you eat and staying with only what you know will do you good. Resist any temptation for a binge because that is an emotional cry from the heart that often hits more in an emotional critical period than any other time.

As the diet progresses, so will your feeling of contentment and well-being. By working with your biorhythms this way, it will help you to create a successful diet regimen – and one that will work. On an intellectually critical day, make sure you don't become forgetful and start nibbling absent-mindedly for this is almost always a clear symptom of any intellectual critical time. On a physical critical day, the strongest desire is to fill the stomach with any (and or all) the food you can lay your hands on.

This is often the time that you feel you have had enough and want to put an end to all this. Be aware and learn to recognise these warning signs. It might seem hard at the time but stay with the diet and it will all get much easier as time passes. Each critical period you get through will help you maintain your new behavioural pattern of eating properly so that you will slim and stay slim.

STOP SMOKING FOR GOOD

Smoking of any kind, at any level, is an addiction and is often closely associated with the way people eat. People tend to put on weight when they first stop smoking, mostly because they tend to nibble more to help fight the body's craving for nicotine. However, you must plan effectively and create a well thought-out campaign to free your system of this craving. From a biorhythmic point of view, this will require a properly timed exercise to ease the problem but you must really want to stop. With the help of biorhythms you can, but it is not all honey and roses.

Make up your chart for at least one month, although two or even three would be much better. Time your start for about two or three days after a positive to negative critical day in the emotional cycle. It is at this time you are unlikely to experience much change in the way you feel and will allow nearly two weeks before the next critical day, when you are most likely to weaken to temptation. Try to be a few days into the early stage of the positive phase of the intellectual rhythm as well but that is not so important. You are better fitted to resist temptation and you should also be physically able to cope and stop smoking.

By the tenth day, around two weeks later you will be expecting your next physical critical day. It ought not to have too much of an effect, especially as it does not last very long. Remember, if you can do it for one day then you can do it for two, then three and so on. After that, a week is nothing and in a month you ought to have stopped with this intelligent use of biorhythms. In the first few days or so of this exercise you will experience a change in your digestive system.

Your body will want more food and drink than usual. If you do eat or drink a little more to compensate, any small weight rise is a part of giving up, so do not worry too much. In addition, and if you feel so inclined, leave your car a little further away from where you are going. If you use public transport then get off the bus or leave the train at an earlier stop. The extra walking involved will all go to help the end result.

HEALTH AND ILLNESS

In recent years, some medical authorities have begun, perhaps a little reluctantly, to acknowledge biorhythms to have some value in health matters. It has been found that the times of certain incubation periods between exposure to, and actually suffering from, a few childhood ailments may correspond with the physical cycle critical days.

Colds and flu seem to tighten their grip on positive to negative physical critical days. It has long been known that people recover more quickly from surgery when in the positive stage of their physical rhythm. And during surgery, bleeding has now been proven to be more profuse on physical critical days.

You should try to make an appointment with your dentist when all three cycles are in the positive phases. When the physical rhythm is in the negative stage you are prone to feel more pain, and not just while visiting the dentist. A fall, a minor injury, a simple ordinary headache, all seem to be more painful at this time. Should the emotional cycle also be in the passive stage, you can make it feel far worse than it actually is because of your current low emotional resistance level.

Heart attacks and strokes occur more when both the physical and sensitivity cycles are critical or in the low phase. It does not follow that this will happen, it is only more likely about to happen when or if you are in poor health.

ACCIDENTS

Accidents occur more frequently on single or multiple critical days because people are likely to feel over-confident. When their rhythms are in the positive phase, just prior to a critical day, they are prone to talk themselves into and out of all kinds of situations. Equally, people tend to misread the signs when they are in their negative stages and do not always take into account all the facts before they commit themselves to a course of action that so easily leads to an incident or an accident.

When this happens, the incident may not cause a physical injury. It could be that a wrong business decision could lead to severe troubles in other ways. One of the main causes of accidents to adults in the home are falls, especially where elderly people are concerned.

Older folk are more prone to falls in the early hours or after a short nap. As people grow older, their metabolism does not come into full play until they have been awake for some time. They should wait a little before attempting to rise, and not make too many sudden moves.

They are more liable to experience a fall on a critical day in their physical cycle more than at any other time, so they should allow time for their autonomic nervous system to become adjusted properly. Much the same goes for children, for they also become prone to accidents in the home on physical rhythm critical days. Equally, it could be as the result of the adult in the home, who may be on an intellectual critical day, who leaves dangerous things lying around unattended.

It is so easy to misjudge things or be forgetful at these times. Do-it-yourself types fall prey to accidents on critical days, as a rule, when their emotional or physical critical days transit from the positive stage to the negative. They are also likely to occur on their positive mini-critical intellectual periods. Many people talk themselves into delusions of adequacy at such times and pay the price later.

The biorhythmic cycles appear to control performance or are at least influential in our main areas of behaviour, that is, physically, emotionally and intellectually. However, it must be stressed that while they have no direct cause and effect in themselves, they are, in each case, subject to the prevailing conditions of the environment of the moment. It has been found that there is a correlation between the state of the individual rhythm and certain factors in our behaviour. More to the point, awareness of the stage or phase of the rhythm allows the individual an opportunity to correct or adjust his or her conduct accordingly. The success rate following such action has always been positive.

Thus, biorhythm cycles are obviously a potential answer to our on and off days, so that the intelligent use and awareness of them ought to be able to provide a more positive approach to life. If, after a short while, you have not experienced any of those unfortunate little incidents and accidents, you will begin to feel far better in yourself.

RELATIONSHIPS

Most of us try to get along as best we can with those around us but it can be difficult at times. In our early childhood, family relationships are very important; they help to shape our basic attitudes and help us form associations with others of the same age as we grow older. When an active youngster has a tantrum on a critical day, it can so easily lead to an accident. At the very least, it will affect the mood of the parents and, should one or both of them not be in a compatible mood, it will lead to domestic disharmony.

Children do not have the developed sense of awareness that most adults should have so, once a parent becomes aware of the effect that biorhythms might have on their children, it is a relatively easy matter for them to plan ahead and allow for such potentially difficult days.

Therefore, if biorhythms can be used to assist a more structured approach to inter-family relationships then parents should have their children's biorhythm chart created. At the very least, it can only lead to a more reasoned response on critical days. Armed with this advanced warning, parents can avoid confrontational, hostile or unproductive moments and be more accommodating at such times.

Parents are not being asked to change their overall attitude but to make small adjustments; to be more understanding not only of themselves but also of their children. This works just as well in reverse. Children will begin to see their parents in a much better light and help them understand that some adults can be reasoned with in times of stress. When we become adults, our relationships are not really that much different, except that we ought to be able to control our moods a little better than when we were children. All relationships are crucial to our lives in one way or another.

Ordinary friendships rely on some kind of compatibility.

When we call in the newsagent's shop for our morning paper and cigarettes, we may indulge in a mild banter, the level of which depends on how well we know each other. At work, associations are more likely to be on the intellectual level – we have to maintain 'face'.

SEX DRIVE

When it comes to love, sex and marriage, we need to be responsive at the right time and be prepared for our partner at the right moment. Our personal sex drive is governed in a cyclic manner in much the same way as any rhythm is and most people think, wrongly, that this is linked with the physical rhythm. Certainly, people are more inclined to feel sexy and are likely to need or have sex when their physical rhythm is in the plus or positive stage than at any other time.

However, if your emotional cycle is in the negative phase, your enjoyment may not be as high and your responses may well be less enthusiastic. If the intellectual rhythm is also negative, 'automatic' sexual activity may upset the partner. On double critical days, your personal response to your physical desire can lead to accidents – caution in more ways than one is strongly advised.

Couples who are actually trying for a child may like to know that the statisticians have found that biorhythms may be linked to the sex of a child. Women seem to have sons more when conception occurs while she is experiencing her physical cycle's positive phase and the negative stage of her emotional rhythm than any other time. More girls tend to be born if conception takes place during the soon-to-be potential mother's low physical cycle and a high emotional cycle.

If both the physical and the emotional cycles are in the positive stage or negative phase together when conception takes place, it is not possible to predict the outcome with any reasonable success.

Pregnant women may like to know that, as their time approaches, they may be able to assess the date and time of the birth of their baby by using their biorhythms. The older the mother-to-be, the more likely the baby will arrive on an intellectual critical day. Ordinary, or natural birth, is more likely to occur when either or both of her physical and her emotional critical days are due.

Should all of the mother's biorhythms be in their positive stages, the birth is often an 'easy' matter but it is much more helpful if her physical biorhythm is positive anyway. On an emotional critical day she is liable to be more worried or tensed up than usual for such an event. This is likely to affect the delivery and make things more difficult.

CHAPTER 10

THE RHYTHMS OF LIFE

Through many a long year, we have proved many times that critical days, especially in the physical cycle, frequently seem to coincide with lowered strength, poor health and, in some extreme cases, even death. Statistically, and for the individuals concerned, these critical or switch-over days have been found to be more accident-prone than non-critical times.

Thus, the obvious watchword has to be caution. As long as the reader bears in mind that biorhythms in themselves are not a cause and effect of anything, in that they do not in themselves make things happen but that they do so often coincide with such problems.

One of the best analogies I can think of is the electric light bulb. Whether or not it has a weak filament, the most likely time for it to 'blow' is as it is switched on or off. It is rare, but not unknown for a bulb to just fail. However, when one is switched on, a burst of power surges through the filament in such a way that, irrespective of its condition, it is just as likely to blow whether it is switched on or off. One moment it pulses with life, the next there is nothing, it is temporarily weakened. Rapidly switching a light bulb on and off in error often has this effect.

ANTICIPATING DANGEROUS PERIODS

Biorhythms may be used to anticipate potentially dangerous periods in your life however healthy you may appear at the time. It does not follow though, that if you have a heart attack or are suffering from a disease that is known to kill, the next critical day will be your last. Nevertheless, whether you are in a hospital or elsewhere, it would be ideal if your biorhythm chart could be displayed at the foot of the bed alongside all the other charts and other paraphernalia used to monitor your progress.

With such information available then, before your critical biorhythmic stages are about to happen, an additional watch could be quite easily be kept on you, just in case. The physical biorhythm is important but so also are the emotional and intellectual rhythms. When faced with difficult decisions, it is important to have a clear mind, unclouded by emotional issues, and free to operate without fear or favour.

Throughout history, lots of awkward, terrible or splendid moments in the lives of many people from all walks of life have depended on their being emotionally free and with an unbiased thought process. However, certain figures from the past, famous or infamous, all made decisions and carried out the deeds they did at either the right or wrong moment as they saw things at the time. But, when we look at their biorhythms, we might now better understand (sometimes) what might have caused them to have taken the actions they did and, more to the point, why they did.

EVA BRAUN

The long-time mistress, companion and, finally, the wife of Adolf Hitler died in the bunker in Berlin alongside her husband of just a few hours sometime during Monday, 30 April 1945. She was born on Tuesday, 6 February 1912, in

Munich. There has been (and still is) much speculation as to whether she was murdered, either by Hitler or an aide loyal to the last, or if she really did commit suicide.

Victims of violence rarely show disturbed biorhythms unless it was their own action that caused their demise. So, if this lady was murdered, the chances are that her biorhythms would have been relatively normal: but if she did take her own life, they would have shown some disturbance.

Her biorhythms for that day were poor. When she married Hitler, she was experiencing an intellectual mini-critical day – the cycle was at absolute nadir. Further, she was approaching a similar position in her physical cycle on the following May Day along with an emotional critical period.

In addition, Eva Braun was an unusual woman who suffered from depression. On the day she died, her biorhythm chart showed how really disturbed she was. She had tried to commit suicide on 1 November 1932 and on looking at her chart for that day, we note her biorhythms to be almost as unbalanced.

Some three years or so after this, she attempted suicide again when yet another one of her moods got the better of her for, on 29 May 1935, Eva Braun tried once again to take her own life. Her biorhythms for the day reflect her emotional and mental state. Her biorhythm chart for the time showed how the day before the attempt she experienced an emotional critical period and the day after she was intellectually critical.

So, with this evidence to hand, when we come to review 30 April 1945, we can probably accept that she probably took her own life. Her biorhythms did not cause her to take her own life but they do reflect the prevailing conditions of her immediate environment at the time. This is just one example of how a figure drawn from history and adjudged, from a biorhythmic point of view, we might see yet another reason for why their thoughts and subsequent actions led them to do what they did.

PRESIDENT JOHN F KENNEDY

It does not always rest with politicians to make decisions that alter a nation's destiny. When Lee Harvey Oswald shot President John F Kennedy on Friday, 22 November 1963, one cannot blame the President for an act that was virtually outside of his control. It was not a direct action of the President himself that caused his own death.

But, when we come to survey his biorhythms for that fateful day there is an interesting conclusion to be reached that has been collated from all the information we now have some 50 years after the event.

These later investigations show that, although Kennedy had been advised of the possibility of an assassination attempt, he chose not to heed the warnings. He was born on 29 May 1917. His biorhythms for that date were up physically and emotionally but at a critical stage in the intellectual cycle. Perhaps he was feeling a tad more confident regarding his popularity as a result. This could have been the reason he decided not to take advantage of a covered, bullet-proof vehicle.

PRESIDENT RONALD REAGAN

Perhaps the best of the modern day United States leaders, Ronald Reagan, was born 6 February 1911 and pursued several careers, first as an actor then as the President of the Screen Actors Guild. For a time, he was the official spokesman for the General Electric Company which led him eventually into politics, initially as a Democrat but he changed later to the Republican side.

He was elected Governor of California where he served two terms. After two failed attempts to become the American leader he was elected President of the United States in 1980 and survived the assignation attempt by John Hinckley a few weeks into his first term on 30 March 1981. He went on to serve a second term in 1984.

He died of pneumonia brought about by complications through Alzheimer's disease on 5 June 2004. He was about to undergo a two day period of critical days in both his emotional and intellectual cycles.

PRESIDENT ABDEL NASSER

President Abdel Nasser Gamel Abdel Nasser died suddenly of a heart attack on Monday, 28 September 1970. He was born on 15 January 1918. At the time of his death, he was about to experience a double critical period in his physical and emotional cycles on the following two days. If he was overdoing things then, his timing was obviously wrong.

The use of biorhythms would have advised him that he was just two days past an intellectual mini-critical period. He was liable to think he could cope with whatever he was given, easily tempted to take on more than usual. With a double-critical period imminent, he was not tempting fate as such, but he would have been well advised to ease off. If he had been aware of his biorhythms, he might have taken a different course of action on that fateful day.

INDIRA GHANDI

Indira Gandhi, the Indian stateswoman and first female Prime Minister of her country, was the daughter of Jawaharlal Nehru, himself a former Prime Minister. Born on 19 November 1917, she became the victim of assassins, members of her own personal Sikh bodyguard, on 31 October 1984.

Her intellectual rhythm was in critical stage, passing from the negative to positive stage. Mrs Gandhi did not always listen to the advice from those who put her interests first. That may have been a contributory cause to her demise.

HAROLD WILSON

Harold Wilson, who was born 11 March 1916, first became British Prime Minister in 1964 and had an interesting political history until his sudden resignation was announced on 16 March 1976. His biorhythms for that day show that he had just experienced a negative to positive physical critical day and that he was on a mini-critical intellectual day in the positive phase.

There seemed no reason for him to step down – and no convincing explanation was ever put forward. However, his wife, Mary, has since said that he always meant to go quite quickly. He had had enough and thought that his memory was failing, suggesting the possible early onset of Alzheimer's. He felt he could no longer do the job in the way that he wanted.

KIM JONG II

Kim Jong II, the one-time leader of North Korea was born on 16 February 1941 and succeeded his father as leader of the country in 1994. It took him some time to become really well established as the supreme head of the country and he finally achieved this after three long years of sheer hard work and patience. He died of a heart attack on 17 December 2011, a few hours before his next physical critical day.

MIKHAIL KALASHNIKOV

Mikhail Kalashnikov, born on 10 November 1919, was both a small arms designer and a long serving Russian General. His name is known (and revered in some places) throughout the world for the various weapons he created, none of which he would admit to as weapons of offence. He always maintained they were weapons of defence. He died in hospital of a stomach haemorrhage on 23 December 2013. All three of his biological rhythms were at absolute nadir.

CLARK GABLE

Clark Gable, the long-time King of Hollywood was born on 1 February 1901, suffered a heart attack on 5 November 1960.

When we look at his biorhythms for this time, we can see that he had just experienced a critical emotional period the day before and, on this day, he was undergoing a physical critical period. He had his second and fatal attack on 16 November 1960, on another physical critical day, but this time he was switching from the positive to the negative phase.

He was also one day away from an emotional critical day, with his intellectual rhythm in negative phase. Obviously, his biorhythms did not cause Gable to die, but their condition was not helpful either and the world lost a much loved and gifted personality.

ALAN LADD

Alan Ladd, another firm and much admired leading Hollywood film favourite was born 3 September 1913 and died suddenly on 29 January 1964. At this time , he was in the middle of a double critical period in his physical and emotional cycles.

He had come to the top of his profession after a rather clever pairing with Veronica Lake – another well-known Hollywood favourite. She was one of the few actresses of her time who was actually smaller than Alan Ladd, which went a long way to help them both appear realistic on screen, and they enjoyed enormous success for a long while.

VERONICA LAKE

Miss Lake was born on 14 November 1922 and died of natural causes on 7 July 1973. Her biorhythms at the time were all at a very low point and she was just 3 days away from a double (emotional/intellectual) critical day.

JUDY GARLAND

Judy Garland was born on 10 June 1922 and died of a drugs overdose on 21 June 1969. Not known for her good health at the best of times toward the end of her life, she was just two days past an intellectual critical day, from positive to negative, and was on an emotional critical day, also positive to negative. She was shortly to experience a physical critical period just three days later on 24 June 1969.

MEL SMITH

Mel Smith, the much loved performer, writer, producer, director and humourist was born on 3 December 1953. He became well known to TV viewers for his work and appearances on Not the Nine O'clock News and Alas, Smith and Jones. He went on to work with Griffith (Griff) Rhys Jones and together they founded what was to become one of the largest TV production companies in the UK. He collapsed early on 19 July 2013 and was declared dead by the ambulance crew. After a post mortem examination, it was made known that he had died of a sudden heart attack.

POPE JOHN-PAUL I

Pope John-Paul I was born Albino Luciani on 17 October 1917 and elected Pope on 26 August 1978. Some 33 days later, late on the evening of 28 September, he allegedly suffered a heart attack and died as a result, but was not found until the very early hours of the following day. Rumours soon abounded suggesting foul play, partly because of his highly original approach to the Papacy in such a short time and also because there was no post mortem.

His biorhythms were quite normal and did not suggest poor health. Given all the circumstances, the accusation that he was poisoned may have had some substance. He was an ordinary, practical man full of common sense. Who knows what political enemies he may have made in so short a time, or what struggles he might have had if he had lived?

MARK SPITZ

Mark Spitz, born 10 February 1950, achieved immortality when he created a still unbeaten record among record-breakers by winning seven gold medals at the 1972 Olympics at the end of August and the beginning of September.

His biorhythms were in a double peak form that must have contributed considerably towards his outstanding success. Between 27 August and 8 September, Spitz won medal after medal, almost within the space of a single week. On 27 August, he had experienced a double critical in the physical and intellectual cycles and another double critical, this time in the physical and emotional cycles, a few days later on 8 September; surely a possible explanation for his enormous success.

NEIL ARMSTRONG

Without a doubt, the most momentous occasion of the last century did not take place here on Earth, but it was a very special Earth man who stepped out on to the surface of the Moon on 20 July 1969. Neil Armstrong, who was born on 5 August 1930, set foot on the Moon with the immortal words: 'That's one small step for a man, one giant leap for mankind.'

He had blasted off on 16 July, on a physically critical day, perhaps an inappropriate day for an event entailing so much physical stress. He then experienced a triple mini-critical day on the 22nd and had to undergo the enormous physical stress of re-entry on the 24th. Despite the phasing of his physical cycle, his two other rhythms were in absolutely peak form for balanced judgement.

Remember also that Armstrong took over the controls to land the lunar module. There could have been no proper dress rehearsal for this but throughout those historic eight days, his rhythms were just about perfect for such a task.

Because of the lack of gravity involved, he would not have needed too much physical strength, except for each end of the journey. However, a razor-sharp mind and emotional balance were essential for a successful mission. Here was something which no other man had ever done before. Just what would happen when he actually landed on the Moon had to be in the realms of pure speculation. In the event, these activities represent the need for perfect biorhythmic timing for what was, perhaps, the most daunting task for any man.

RONNIE BIGGS

Ronnie Biggs was a villain all his adult life and became almost revered for his (small) part in the Great Train Robbery of 1963 when he was asked to recruit a substitute driver for the train. He was caught because his finger prints were found on a used sauce bottle. He was subsequently arrested, put on trial and sent to prison for 30 years in 1964.

He served around 15 months and was helped to escape in 1965 and he spent the next 36 years a free but hunted man. He surrendered to the English authorities in 2001 and was sent back to prison but released in 2009 because of poor health. When he died on 18 December 2013 he was about to endure an emotional critical day with his physical and intellectual cycles at their nadir.

CLAUDIO ABBADO

The world famous pianist, musician and conductor born 26 June 1933 and died 20 January 2014, after a long illness. He had been operated on for stomach cancer at the turn of the century. When he died, he was experiencing a double critical day. His physical cycle was changing from positive to negative while his emotional cycle was changing from negative to positive. His intellectual cycle was at the lowest point of the rhythm.

IS THIS YOUR DAY?

Remember, such conditions tends to last only for one day but there are a few occasions when some of the combinations can affect an individual for 24 hours – or even more in some circumstances. As a rule, this tends to happen more with the plus or positive stages than with the negative periods.

This would be a good time to create your personal biorhythm chart so that you can be ready to make the simple adjustments necessary to help better control your affairs. All the information you need to set up your personal biogram together with the interpretative material to help you make the right decisions are here in this book.

Furthermore, once you have set up your chart, you can also travel back in time to when you made certain decisions and acted the way you did. Indeed, once you have the birth date of anyone, those close to you, your idols or even people from the past, it becomes possible to assess their biorhythms for whatever purpose. This may well help to give you some if not all of the answers as to why they made the decisions they did or acted in the way that they did.

Either way, looking ahead, it never hurts to plan and prepare properly for those special times when that little bit of extra attention to detail can make all the difference between success or failure.

CHAPTER 11

THE RHYTHMS OF NATURE

There is an all pervading rhythm to life and nature. Rhythms and cycles feature dominantly, not only in the biological study of man and his behavioural patterns or even in the history of the race, but also in practically everything else that we care to investigate.

There are ultradian cycles, that is, rhythms of less than 24 hours duration, circadian rhythms, or those of around 24 hours length and infradian rhythms which last a lot longer, perhaps to as much as a year or more in some cases.

The study of cycles is fascinating and certainly deserves a mention here because there are such a wide variety of rhythms that the average man has probably never really considered or perhaps, has never heard of in some cases. The strange thing here is that they do affect him or her in some way or another, more or less every day of their life, whether asleep or awake.

In each case, these are documented studies either proven under proper laboratory conditions or, where possible, observed in the natural state. As this particular chapter is about men and women and their behavioural patterns, we will start with them. Where we speak of men we also include women unless we specifically state otherwise.

'NIGHT' AND 'MORNING' PEOPLE

Apart from sleep patterns which, under normal circumstances, take place once a day, usually at night when all natural diurnal life rests, man shows a definite rhythmic pattern in every aspect of his life.

The human body temperature reaches a peak during waking hours and is at its lowest point when you are asleep. As your temperature rises, so does your efficiency; conversely, you become far less effective as your temperature drops. None of us are exactly alike for we all respond to our body rhythms as individuals, not collectively.

This why some of us may be considered as 'night' or 'morning' people or perhaps, more popularly, as 'owls' or 'larks'. Almost all animals sleep or, more correctly, have to sleep to survive. And still, after all this time, nobody is really sure why, except that in every animal and human one reason is to rest and restore the status quo and overall balance of health physically, emotionally and intellectually. Elsewhere, all theories about sleep and what it is for are still largely that, theories.

Perhaps the best reason given to date is that it is time for the body to restore itself after all the exercise it receives, wanted or otherwise, while we are awake.

Most of us sleep for an average period of anywhere between seven and nine hours a day. These people tend to live slightly longer than those who disrupt their normal sleep patterns through shift work or for other reasons. When the ordinary pattern of life is disrupted in this fashion, such folk may experience weaker health trends and die younger, partly due to this. Another danger for people who experience a loss of sleep is fatigue which often leads to accidents.

Those who sleep well seem to worry less and can take most things in their stride. So, a good, sound sleep may have something to do with our learning processes. One thing is for sure, we need a normal sleep pattern: it must suit us personally, and it must be regular. There is a very strong sleep drive in young adults which lessens or weakens in most of us as we grow older. Elderly people do not need as much sleep as the young and they should allow for this and adjust their days accordingly. However, whatever their personal sleep pattern is, at whatever age, they will still be an 'owl' or a 'lark'.

One way of checking which of these two categories applies to you would be to take your temperature on the hour every hour until you go to bed, a task that would have to be spread over several weeks to be anything like an accurate survey. If, as you do this, you keep a graph of the readings, it becomes easier to judge your most effective periods, so that you could make simple adjustments to your way of life. By timing your maximum efforts to coincide with the periods of the highest readings, you would increase your personal efficiency that much more.

Everyone has a natural eating rhythm, although most people tend to ignore this because of their social or business obligations. We have already noticed that it would be better for some folk to take in sustenance of some kind every ninety minutes, for instance, while others tend to benefit more from three main meals a day – with nothing in between.

The constituent parts of any meal affects our efficiency in such different ways. While some eat hearty breakfasts with a couple of meals later in the day, others get much more from a light snack first thing with a heavier meal mid-morning.

The composition and timing of such a regimen needs to be adjusted to individual requirements so, if you feel you might benefit from such an experiment, go ahead. You will become more efficient and feel a lot better in yourself. Additionally, you might inherit a better sleep pattern as well.

LIFE STATISTICS

On average, your heart beats 103,680 times a day and, of course, this organ is a part of another cycle, the vascular system. The heart pumps blood around your body in a never ending cycle that has detectable variations in much the same way as do your sleep cycles, feeding habits or other bodily functions.

For as long as your heart continues to beat, you will, on an average day breathe 24,000 times, drink about 1.7 litres (about 3 pints) of varying liquids, consume an average 6.6 kilos (about 3lbs) of food and walk approximately 3.5 kilometres (about 2 miles) using some 750 muscles in the process.

Also during this period, you may speak about 4,800 words and, as well as doing all these other things, you will utilise about 7,000,000 brain cells. In the meantime, your hair will grow about 0.04 cm (around 0.017 inches), your fingernails grow about 0.000046 inches and your toenails will grow some 0.000031 inches. And all that is in just a 24 hour period. Your body clock has many other cycles during this one day period that can positively stagger anyone who is unaware of how his or her body functions.

In this relatively new science of chrono-biology, many discoveries have been made about our bodies and the cycles and rhythms to which we are subjected. Irrespective of the biorhythmic behavioural cycles and periods, we can actually plan out a day and time certain activities almost to the hour for best effect.

For example, if out driving at night, our sight is at its weakest point at about 02:00 hours and our lowest ebb altogether is between 04:00 and 05:00 hours. We make the most errors between 03:00 and 04:00 hours in the morning, which might make some of us wonder why so many babies choose to arrive anywhere between midnight and 04:00 hours.

Men tend to respond more to their sex drive between 07:00 and 08:00 hours in the morning because, while both sexes produce more sex hormones at this hour than at any other time in the day, it does rather depend on whether you are an 'owl' or a 'lark' as to how, or if, you respond to this particular drive. Despite this, we are at our most creative in the morning between 10:00 and 12:00 hours and our digestion is at its peak around 13:00 hours.

We are best at sport between 13:00 and 14:00 hours and are more adept at dealing with problems between 15:00 and 16:00 hours. Shortly after 16:00 hours, our bodies tend to take off again and we perform very well at our 'hobby' sports – cricket, football, jogging or rugby, etc.

Our sense of taste, hearing and smell are much more acute during this period, which is why so many of both sexes prefer to socialise, dine and then make love up to about 22:00 hours in the evening – whether they are an 'owl' or a 'lark'.

Between then and midnight we all slow down a little, some more quickly than others, ready for the sleep period we all know we must have and cannot do without if we are to face the following day in much the same way – and so on and so on.

If married, you will probably make love about 3,000 times and spend a total time equal to fourteen years working. 20 to 24 years spent in bed is the norm. Travelling takes care of five years while dressing, washing, shaving or applying make-up will account for another four years. You will probably spend as much as 70 days just preening yourself and looking in the mirror.

If you are a smoker, you may well consume almost a quarter of a ton (over 1200 kilos) of tobacco. The average intake of food in the course of a normal life span, when taken as a whole, is also quite staggering. This is probably because under normal circumstances we tend to think of just one meal at a time.

During a total period of six years just spent eating, the average person will consume 6,000 loaves of bread, 10,000 eggs, 8,811 kilos of butter and 44,053 kilos of fruit and vegetables. This will be washed down with some 90,920 litres of a wide variety of liquids.

Man's sweet tooth will dispose of 17,621 kilos of sugar while he will eat about 50 head of cattle and some 300 chickens. Shopping for all of that food, along with everything else as well will take about three years of waiting in queues. And not content merely to delve into all our physical idiosyncrasies and all of our senses, scientists have made other discoveries in their search for cycles and rhythms.

OCCUPATIONAL CYCLES

Loosely using birthdates as the criteria, it has been discovered that occupations are high on the agenda of cyclic performance. It has been found that musicians, for example, have a better chance of success when born during November, January or February, than at any other time.

This is not to imply that during the low period, August in this case, there is little chance of becoming successful in this field. Architects flourish better if born during December, May and June; their low point is September or October.

Bankers seem to do so much better when born during in August than those born in March. If born during October you have a better than average chance of becoming a successful journalist or editor than if born in December.

Cyclic performance is noted and logged over such long periods of time that, after a while, it seems that even some of the occupations here may be subject to a rhythm within a rhythm. This is true to such an extent that it is virtually possible to predict certain phenomena with a more than average chance of success. Not only that, it also appears that other cyclic events are closely linked, even when they share no other relationships that can be detected or determined at the time.

WHEELS WITHIN WHEELS

It might be difficult to accept that there seems to be a link between police states and temperature fluctuations that, in turn, can affect patterns of style in the world of art. Co-operation and the integration of views apparently fall into the same pattern as the phenomenon of war, crop improvements and palace intrigues. All these events have been found to operate in a world-wide 100 year cycle, itself a periodic phenomenon.

While the atmosphere in which we live varies slightly throughout the world from country to country and from area to area within a country, the surface air pressure at sea level is, on average, about 65.4N (or around 14.7 pounds per square inch), about one ton per square foot.

This pressure is measured by a barometer and recorded as inches of Mercury. Thus, 65.4N (14.7 pounds per square inch) at sea level equals 29.91 of Mercury. This barometric pressure is affected by, and changes with, the climate and can move up or down according to the state of the weather.

A rising barometer is an indication of high pressure on the way and this is associated with fine dry spells, as a rule. A falling barometer indicates poor weather: rain, winds and storms. After long years of study, it has been found that barometric pressure has moved in a rhythmic pattern of 7.6 years. Changes of pressure seem to influence man and his moods and, in turn, he reflects these moods in many ways.

A falling barometer can produce, or is associated with, symptoms of irritability, forgetfulness and restlessness. There are also regular bouts of sleeplessness recorded at this time, and all of these negative attitudes have been proved to be related in some way to road traffic and industrial accidents. Suicides have also been found to occur more during this same period. The falling barometer is almost always a sign of some danger and there have been studies that have proved a definite correspondence between human behavioural patterns and weather variations both in the short period and the long.

Over 100 year periods it has been shown that during dry and cold spells, people tend to rebel against the accepted order of things in cyclic spells. Individualism, race pride and civil wars tend to occur more often.

In the wet and warm spells, people seem to be quite co-operative, more willing to listen to each other and to become more organised. In dry and warm periods, democracy slowly begins to suffer at all levels, from state control at government height, through to local social life; personal freedoms tend to decline.

There may be more business aggression but financial confidence tends to decline and there may be economic depression. In cold and wet periods, there is a gradual de-centralisation of government, people need, want and strive for more individualistic self-expression. But the more freedom is pursued, the more likely the whole balance of things is likely to collapse once more and anarchy begins to take over prior to the next weather spell.

It is not quite as straightforward and simplistic as this but, a check on weather conditions during a 100 year period will show how much of what has been described here does occur and it all happens in almost pre-determined cycles. Local crime occurs in patterns and may be linked with the weather variation. During summer, July and August, rape, serious assault and murders peak, these more especially so between the hours of 18:00 hours (6 o'clock at night) to 06:00 hours (6 o'clock in the morning).

The crime of burglary, however, is more likely to occur between 18:00 hours through to 02:00 hours (6 o'clock in the evening) and 02:00 hours (2 o'clock in the morning) Saturday night between late November and the end of February. June sees an upsurge of admissions to mental hospitals and suicide attempts. Curiously, it is also the month in which more marriages usually take place...

In the USA between 1920 and 1955, a clearly defined pattern was observed in the construction of residential buildings. This cycle apparently exhibited a 33-month periodicity. But what is really fascinating about such cyclic events is why they ever occur in the first place and where do we start to look for the root cause?

We know very little about our discoveries in these areas but we do know, for example, that there is a definite cycle governing the abundance of snowshoe rabbits in Canada with a length of 9.6 years. The lynx, hawk, owl and marten populations have the same cycle but we do not know what the cause of the cycle may be. In the last 3-400 years or so, scientists and researchers have been finding rhythms and cycles galore.

Some of these have been discovered by accident, a few by design where the researchers have realised that 'something' was there and started to search for it. We may be discovering, or re-discovering a lost art or science – we simply do not know.

Certain historical patterns repeat themselves, both in the same country and in other parts of the world. The events seem to be closely similar to what has gone before.

COSMIC CYCLES

Beyond the bounds of earthly ties are the mysterious forces that compel the Universe in its constant cyclic performance.

We are able to predict these rhythmic motions with tremendous accuracy, but can only hazard guesses as to their cause. We have also come to accept that with so much interdependence between these rhythms and cycles, if one should fail, unknown forces can be unleashed.

If, one day, the Moon should fail to rise, for instance, would the tidal system here on Earth fail to turn as well? What would happen if the length of a day suddenly altered noticeably? As a matter of fact, the length of our day has altered, just perceptibly about 25 years ago. But the real effect, if any, will not be noticed for quite a few million years yet.

You may smile and think there is nothing to worry about now, but suppose this is part of a hitherto undiscovered cycle which does have some kind of an effect now?

The recent onset of the many weather extremes, the storms, heat waves and dry spells that have been occurring all over the world, some in places that have never experienced anything like them in local living or recorded memory.

What has caused them? We simply do not know – yet. We can only guess at some of the answers or give part answers – now. In later years, we may find some or all of the answers and then be ready for the phenomenon next time, if there is a next time. One day, someone is going to find the key. It could be tomorrow, it may be ten or a hundred years from now.

In the meantime, inexplicably, we discover mouse plagues occur in four year cycles and every commodity price we have studied also fluctuates in cycles. The number of babies born each day occurs in cycles, glaciers are known to melt in cycles and the amount of cheese we eat fluctuates in cycles.

SYNCHRONICITY

One fundamental fact of similar cyclic performances that has come to light is the astonishing synchronicity with which everything all tends to interact. All cycles with the same duration actually peak and trough at the same time. This provides evidence of something that we do not yet understand at this stage, even if we do appreciate that it can no longer be classified as random behaviour. There are over 30 widely differing events that fall into an eight-year cycle which has been studied over a prolonged period from the mid 1780's to the mid 1960's. In each case, they reached their high and low spots at the same time during this period.

Cigarette production from 1880; lead production from 1821; red squirrel abundance from 1926; pig-iron prices from 1784; sugar prices over more than a 200 year period; and the growth of pine trees from about 1770. Some patterns are also repeated in cycles that are not of eight years' duration.

Some are 5.91 years long, some are of 9.6 years, while others are 11.2 years in duration. There are mysterious forces at work. This fairly new study of cycles and rhythms could one day allow us to predict far more accurately that ever before our own potential destiny.

It opens new areas of thought with which we may merely play at present. Not that we necessarily understand this new toy we have found. We are not even sure that we have a toy, or that we have the whole toy.

It may only be a part of it, like a single piece of track from a model railway set. This is an age of discoveries, far more than the early part of the 20th century ever was. And the speed with which we are travelling suggests possible answers just around the corner, or the next one, or the next one...

CHAPTER 12

THE INTUITIONAL CYCLE AND OTHER RHYTHMS

We have shown that each of the three major rhythms have three critical or change points. The first occurs at the start with the second at the halfway stage, when it changes from positive to negative, and the third happens at the end of the cycle, which is also the start of the next positive phase.

The physical cycle critical or change days occur on day 1, 12 and 23 while in the emotional cycle they happen on day 1, 15 and 28. In the intellectual rhythm they take place on day 1, 17 and 33. In the intuitional cycle they take place on day 1, 18 and 38.

Generally speaking, it is best to allow at least 24-36 hours for any effect to establish itself or until that particular period has passed in any of the cycles. This is rather much in the same way you would an approaching, exact and departing aspect in astrology.

When in the first or positive part of a cycle, you will feel much more alert, emotionally responsive and perceptive. In the second or negative phase of a rhythm, you feel less responsive, alert and perceptive. On a critical day, when the phase of the cycle changes, you may become error prone.

Your thinking can become clouded, judgement is faulty and unreliable, accidents can happen. It would be best to defer important matters because you are likely to feel uncooperative and make the wrong decisions. If it is possible, you should try to avoid physically overdoing things and not let trivia get you down.

Here would be a good time to make the reader aware of other cycles that biorhythm experts have and studied, and are still.

Of all the other rhythms, there is a rather largely unknown cycle of some 38 days that appears to influence our intuitional, sixth sense, or 'inner ability' to successfully think things through without any logical reasoning behind what we do. This particular rhythm will be of special interest to those many people who work or use their intuitive abilities. Members of the various police forces, the emergency services and those employed in similar occupations come immediately to mind because this cycle does seem to have some kind of an effect where natural prescience is concerned.

As you are now more aware, biorhythms are a major part of the much larger study of Chrono-biology. The three main cycles are continuous measurable physiological changes said to influence human behaviour patterns in the physical, emotional and intellectual senses. When you are aware of them, they help you to plan your life much more effectively.

It is important that you are aware that the three main cycles, the physical, the emotional or sensitivity and the intellectual, irrespective of their individual or collective phases, do not have any direct or apparent cause and effect but it does seem that they do exert some kind of influence.

THE INTUITIONAL CYCLE

We have been aware of a possibly rather useful but relatively unknown cycle of 38 days for some time and it appears to hold sway over our intuitional abilities.

THE INTUITIONAL CYCLE AND OTHER RHYTHMS

Like the three principal rhythms, this cycle has its first critical or change days at its beginning, at the halfway stage when it changes from positive to negative, and at the end of the cycle, which is also the start of the next positive phase. Collectively, these are days 1, 19 and 38.

Generally speaking, it is best to allow at least 24-36 hours for any effect to establish itself or until it has passed, much as in any of the cycles. This is much in the same way as you might be advised in respect of an approaching, exact or a departing aspect in astrology.

When in the first or positive part of any cycle, you will feel much more alert, emotionally responsive and perceptive. In the second or negative phase of a rhythm, you feel less responsive, alert and perceptive. On a critical day, when the phase of the cycle changes, you may become error prone.

Your thinking can become clouded, judgement is faulty and unreliable, accidents can happen. It would be best to defer important matters because you are likely to feel uncooperative and make the wrong decisions. If it is possible you should try to avoid physically overdoing things and not let trivia get you down.

A lot of people who have studied the Intuitional rhythm have been striving to achieve an understanding of which of our senses it appears to govern and they have arrived at some sort of agreement on the possible behaviour patterns the rhythm might yield.

When in the first or positive part of this rhythm, the subject seems to be very much 'aware' that their perception rate and ability to 'read' others and or their intentions is heightened. They seem to 'know' how events may turn out and their 'hunches' so often prove to be right – in spite of what the 'facts' may say at the time. Somehow, the real thoughts and ideas of those who are around them are easier to fathom out.

When in the second half, or the negative phase of the cycle, these abilities are considerably lessened. Most people who so often rely on their ability here tend to find that this natural talent for such things becomes somewhat blunted. We are much less perceptive and unsure of what or when to do anything for the best.

When the intuitional cycle is in this phase, the individual should learn to rely more on what he or she actually knows rather than on what they may think they know. The ability to 'perceive' what might be behind the actions of another is somewhat dulled.

On the critical days of this cycle, such apparently natural judgement becomes very unreliable. People ought to disregard what hunches they think they might have because, quite simply, they are prone to making mistakes.

Incidents and accidents are liable to occur, so people would be best advised to delay or defer anything they might regard as specifically important to them at the time. This particular cycle has been studied for some time now and it really merits a much better status than it has actually been given so far. This is largely because it has been neglected on the grounds that we have had rather little information on which to base our theories. However, what is written here will give the reader a good basis with which he or she may experiment as they see fit because it is all based on research work.

CALCULATION OF THE INTUITIONAL CYCLE

To discover the present state of your personal intuition rhythm, divide the amount of days you have been alive by 38. Multiply the remainder by 38 and the result will be your present state. A full explanation of how to do this will be found in the chapter on calculations.

In the first half of this cycle, the 'mini-critical' day is on day nine, when the cycle peaks. Little passes you by as you somehow manage to circumvent all the facts as others may see them and get to the crux of the matter without too much effort because your innate sixth sense is at its height.

In the second half, or negative phase of the rhythm, this ability is lessened, your innate feelings for such things are blunted and you are less perceptive, unsure of what to do or which way you should turn for the best.

On a critical day, as the cycle changes from one level to another, your inherent natural judgment is faulty or unreliable, so it would be best to disregard hunches. You might be error prone, accidents may happen and you should put off important decisions, if at all possible.

When the intuitional cycle is at its lowest point on day 29, it is better for you not to rely on anything but the facts as you see them. Follow any hunches by all means but be aware that it could cost you if you don't think things through as you should at such a time.

OTHER CYCLES AND RHYTHMS

It is overwhelmingly recognised as well as understood by the majority of those who work in the world of chrono-biology, psychology and science in general, that we all have a very wide range of natural cycles and rhythms that are known to fluctuate through all of us each day and night.

There are a few people, a mere handful perhaps, who do not or may not seem to respond or recognise the influence of these phenomena. In addition, there are even less who appear to remain on an even keel throughout their day and who show little, if any, evidence of any type of behaviour pattern at all. Somehow, these folk exhibit the same behavioural patterns all day and every day. In spite of this sort of behaviour, we will now try to illustrate how the rest of us do show a certain pattern of behaviour in the way we respond in a general way to these cycles – usually without realising it.

What little (mostly) unconscious responses that we do exhibit show that we seem to have at least an inner understanding of our rhythms and that the adjustments we make consciously or otherwise during the course of our individual working tasks and schedules help us tremendously.

But this is made more curious because, while we seem to be aware or attuned to them, we generally strive to minimise any potential or actual stress in both our working environment and our social lives. Over and above all this and, generally speaking of course, the peaks and troughs of our daily lives are experienced by us all in the following 24 hour periods. This has nothing to do with our normal biorhythmic state but how we tend to react at these particular times and days.

We will start the survey of a typical day with an eight o'clock call.

MORNINGS
08:00 to 10:30

Our energy levels are high as is the level of our alertness, stamina and strength. For most people, this is usually the best time to plan important meetings, to schedule and or begin new projects, write letters and or return phone calls. It is really the best time to meet with important people and that includes both clients and fellow employees partly because between nine and ten o'clock, we tend to give and receive our most firm handshake when meeting with new faces. The firmer a handshake may feel, the more responsive we are inclined to be toward that individual, irrespective of his or her position within or outside of the company for whom we work.

Once you appreciate, realise and accept how important this particular peak period can be, try not to waste it on mundane or simple tasks. In another field altogether, this is the best time to have a doctor's appointment especially if we are to have an injection, for around nine o'clock is the least painful time for it.

10:30 to the LUNCH HOUR
Any feeling of being 'with-it' or your 'go-getting' talents may well have begun to pall by now. During these two or three hours or so, your energy levels start to lag somewhat, resulting in less physical stamina and or mental alertness. Ideally, this is one of the best moments to take a coffee break and mull over long-term plans.

However, now is also one of the best times of the day to think through any basic ideas for any future strategies or for getting material ready for a business or a social meeting. Return phone calls or send emails if you failed to do so earlier. This can be one of the most creative periods of any day and is, curiously, a most effective period for attending a job interview.

AFTERNOONS
LUNCH TIME to around 15:00 HOURS
By now you will have had your fill according to your individual needs because your digestive system is at its peak. You will begin to come on strong again.

The personal energy levels of most folk begin to peak again because, after stopping and eating, many of us seem to regain that all important initial impetus. This is a particularly good time for taking part in sporting events, competitive or otherwise.

What may have been good in the morning hours will be of excellent use now for both your physical stamina and mental alertness will be at a high rating again. This is a marvellous time for getting involved in essential work and is excellent for first discussing and making difficult decisions or, perhaps, having meetings with clients.

15:00 HOURS to around 16:30 HOURS

While the momentum of the day is carrying you along you may experience a quite natural biological lowering in your body's blood sugar level. At about 16:00 hours, people tend to feel themselves slow down as their stamina and mental acuity begins to ease off somewhat.

Around now is a good time to have another tea or coffee break, or even enjoy a small snack of some kind. One should go over all or any plans made earlier or for paying attention to on-going tasks and projects or for carrying out simple run-of-the-mill basic research work.

AFTER 16:30 HOURS

Many of us may now have to turn to pressing demands like deadlines, for example. More people than ever find this short period is when they seem to experience stress and urgency more than at any other time of the day. In turn, this often leads to worrying moments inwardly. We may also feel anxiety lurking not far away because we feel there is a lot to do with only a short amount of time to do it in.

If possible, now is the time to take a quick walk around the workplace area for this does help to steady the nerves and clear the mind. If it is at all possible, a jog out in the open air would do you the world of good for this is the best time for that kind of exercise. This all fits in nicely with our general well-being and growth overall. Curiously, it is about now that our nails and hair grow the fastest.

EVENING HOURS

Between now and bed time, the evening meal period can vary enormously. It is very much up to the individual person and the demands on their time. Those who have to work through what might be their normal time for an evening meal often have to force themselves to work on.

Between five o'clock and seven o'clock, your sense of taste, smell and hearing are at your most acute. But the hectic pace of today's business environment can often demand that we should keep working through well past this time without stopping for any sustenance.

To remain at whatever peak you do manage to sustain, you should try to find the time to take a short rest period. If nothing else, take the time to help you re-charge your batteries with a tea or a coffee for this will work wonders for you. Be aware, this is not the time for alcohol. Any short spell of relaxation taken around now can and does work wonders but do avoid any alcoholic drink. This short stop goes a long way to help maintain your physical energy and mental alertness to stay more positive for a few hours longer.

After six o'clock and for the rest of the evening hours may be when most people tend to imbibe alcohol for this is usually when the liver works at its peak. For most of us, between now and ten o'clock in the evening is our best time for being with other people in a business or formal sense, romantically or just for the social company.

NIGHT HOURS

Most people tend to go to bed any time from around ten to ten-thirty at night, through to midnight. It is mostly habit, although many of us tend to vary our closing down times for all sorts of reasons. Our sleep patterns work in a rhythmic form as well. For most of us, this will be a ninety minute cycle that lasts in one of three phases. These will be light sleep, deep sleep or rapid eye movement (R.E.M.) periods.

Should you be awakened accidentally or deliberately during an REM period, then later you will almost certainly go about your affairs tired out and quite bad-tempered. When you suddenly come out of a deep sleep period in this manner, the effect is more heightened and you are likely to remain unfeeling and unbalanced for a lot longer. However, should you awaken from a light sleep period, you will feel refreshed and ready for the challenge of the day.

If you are a night worker, you are most likely to be at your lowest ebb at around 02:00 hours, especially if you are driving. This goes for any vehicle you take on the road because this is when your eyes are at their lowest point of focus.

Eyes can and often do fail to focus for long periods at almost any time around now. A little later on and until around 04:00 hours, is when we are likely to be well out of kilter and become accident prone. Between now and 05:00 hours is our lowest point throughout the whole day. As a mere man, it is a constant wonder to me why it is so many babies arrive between midnight and now. As to how the ladies manage to cope with all this extra strain has always been beyond me.

DAYS OF THE WEEK

Much of what has been described may be tempered by which day of the week it is. A great deal of effort and energy has been put into a lot of research into the way we are inclined to behave on certain days of the week, which makes these extra few notes prove to be very helpful.

MONDAY

Try not to arrange anything for a Monday morning unless you must. Most of us tend to live to a 24-hour clock while, in essence, our bodies lean more toward a 25-hour time style. Our usual weekend existence tends to affect this and, come Monday morning, we are likely to be more out of sync than on any other day. Energy levels are quite likely to be low. Our concentration levels are not all that reliable either. For the majority of us, it often proves wiser to spend the day reasonably quietly to catch up with things gradually.

TUESDAY

Tuesday is one of our better days, especially the morning hours. Today has been shown to be the best day of the week on which to begin almost any or all health regimes. Now, this is most encouraging for all of you trying to lose weight or start a diet. But remember, not to rush in to get something like this under way because if you do, it isn't likely to last very long.

WEDNESDAY

Wednesday can come as a culture shock for many. One should avoid keep-fit classes like the plague. Do your best to stay out of office or factory floor cliques but do try to join in some sort of social life after work in the p.m. hours. Quite a few folk tend to feel rather low all day. The previous weekend is now dead and buried and with it all the fun and excitement of the period. The next weekend is a tad too far away to look forward to, so make the most of this day while you can.

THURSDAY

Thursday favours a few activities that should really surprise you and none of them are linked. Thursday morning is almost perfect for making love, especially in the a.m. hours, shortly after you have woken up. Both men and women have proved to be at their most responsive at this time and especially on this day.

In addition to this, most managers, and that includes the boss, tend to be less aggressive, so now is the time to make (sensible) suggestions regarding the work load or other matters because these people tend to be far more flexible in their outlook at this time. Thursday is also the best day of the week to apply for promotion or to ask for a raise, but don't expect answers the same day.

FRIDAY

Friday, however, seems to be the best day for all other money matters. This is the best day to invest, save, make arrangements for loans or negotiate deals involving money. People who deal in money are often more relaxed during the Friday morning hours probably because the weekend is beckoning and they want to be away and out of it. Curiously, this evening is also the night to drink rather more freely than usual, although your sleep patterns will suffer if you overdo it.

SATURDAY

Saturday is the best day for any keep-fit regime, working in the garden or being busy within the home. Using all our different muscles and not having to think in our usually regimented five–days at work helps us all to loosen up.

SUNDAY

Sunday really does deserve to be called a day of rest. All our usual daily tasks should have been completed, certainly by noon but, because we now have more time on our hands, couples are more likely to argue on this day than on any other. Men tend to be more easy-going or relaxed than the ladies.

Despite your personal daily biorhythms, these activities and the times that they are liable to exert their full strengths are well worth knowing about, especially if or when you use this knowledge to capitalise on the strengths and weaknesses of others. Currently, only the three physical, emotional and intellectual rhythms are used in compatibility assessments.

Up to and until recently, there simply hasn't been enough data in respect of our knowledge of the intuition rhythm as there is now. The compatibility shown earlier now has a fourth cycle to which we may refer. It is only natural that any research work has to be fairly slow because of the nature of the subject and the amount of people involved. However, what we have learned and know so far is encouraging.

People do respond to their intuition much more than was first appreciated. It has only been with the help of those folk who didn't mind admitting that they felt their intuition was helpful and that they used it could we begin to progress. I have created and attached a four-rhythm compatibility assessment table to which people may refer for their study and perusal as they see fit.

OTHER RHYTHMS

Biorhythms 'came to life' again in the middle 1970s and while it has been (very) slow-going in the UK, in other countries much has been achieved. Other cycles and rhythms have been discovered but there is even less really known or understood about them yet.

A so-called 'mastery' rhythm has been created by combining the physical and intellectual cycles together.

Those who have promoted this idea claim that it allows for the ability of the individual to take command and control of any situation he or she may find themselves in. It seems to work with some people but I have found that it does not seem to affect all people.

Also mentioned is a 'wisdom' cycle which has been created from an assessment of the emotional and intellectual rhythms together. This is said to enhance the subject's ability to more fully comprehend matters that may not normally be that clear to him or her. This is still under review and, like the 'mastery' cycle, it has not yet received sufficient support to say if the efficacy claimed is good one way or the other.

With these two relatively unknown ideas comes the so-called 'passion' rhythm which is a combination of the physical and emotional cycles. This allegedly creates a whole new and strong desire in the individual to pursue more avidly something or someone that has taken their fancy at the time. Please feel free to test these ideas for yourself.

There are two more suggestions that are under review in various areas. One is known as the 'aesthetic' cycle which is virtually self-explanatory. It should be regarded as a cycle on its own and has a total period of some 48 days. The first critical day is on day one, the second being experienced at day 24 and the third comes on the last day which should also be regarded as the first day of the next positive phase, et al. People who have or who are experimenting with this rhythm suggest one should allow at least 48 hours for the effect of these days to pass.

There is also alleged to be a 'spiritual' rhythm in which the person concerned may feel or become more involved in religious matters. The period allowed for this 53 days with the first critical day being experienced on day 1, the second comes on day 26 or 27. As with all the other cycles, the last day of this cycle should also be regarded as the first day of the next positive period. It is also best to allow at least 48 hours to pass in respect of the critical days for this cycle.

These last five ideas are offered and recorded in conjunction with the three main cycles so that one may assess them as they look at the principal reason for wanting such information.

There are couple of programs covering these ideas to be found on the Internet but please be aware of the claims of program promoters.

CHAPTER 13

THE SPORTING WORLD

Most of us flourish best at one sport or another, either as an amateur or professionally at around 13:00 hours but this tendency passes after about an hour or so and by around 14:30 hours, what prowess we might show tends to ease up. However, this is not so much for the professionals because they train or are trained to last much longer and not necessarily through the hours mentioned.

Nevertheless, having said that, after a couple of hours of apparent 'rest', our abilities at sporting activities take off again and we are able to perform very well at what might be termed our 'hobby sport'. This would mean activities such as football, jogging, rugby, cricket, golf and tennis or even darts and table-tennis.

To be successful at any sporting event, outdoors or indoors, you should be aware of your individual biorhythm stages at all times. Of course, much depends with which sport you are involved. The best time to prepare or train for your particular activity is usually during the p.m. hours, although it is recognised that there are some sporting people who have to train much earlier than this, for a variety of reasons.

This would be a good time to remind you to re-read the chapter that explains the nature of people who are either 'larks' or 'owls', that is, those who either prefer the early part of the day or those who come alive during the later hours.

For example, 'owls' rarely achieve much in the early hours when it comes to golf, but as the day wears on, their skills soon come to their rescue. Few golfers train in the early hours, although there is nearly always someone who will be out at first light trying to perfect their play. However, having said that, there are probably just as many amateur golfers who like to get on a course around 08:00 hours partly because they enjoy the pleasure of not only being in the open air but also for the game.

Golf primarily requires good visual skills. It is good for your health and as there are quite a few miles for a player to clock up, he or she will need good physical fitness and a fair degree of social skill to help them succeed. This game is often the way for people to enjoy a get-together or meet someone new for the first time. It is also one of these rare activities where you will either have to have or will need to develop a sense of community connections.

As a rule, the best time for golfers to compete would be when their cycles are in the positive stage for, biorhythmically speaking, statistics have shown this to be the case with the vast majority of competition winners over the years. Like most athletes, especially those who take part in stadium based competitions, critical days do not appear to matter a great deal. Such folk either win in great glory or lose out in abject failure.

Boxers, however, seem to do quite well when their physical and intellectual cycles are on a high level. Boxing relies naturally on the amount of physical stamina present more than anything else but the ability to perceive when and where to strike effectively suggests the need for intellectual ability as well. Thus, to ensure that little extra plus a boxer's biorhythms should be at a high point in all three cycles.

Generally speaking, however, statistics show most boxers do well when their emotional and intellectual cycles are high and their physical rhythm is in the negative phase ascending toward the next critical day. Boxers should never compete against each other when any of their cycles, especially the physical rhythm, is at a critical stage.

Swimming is not too dissimilar to running but is mainly for those who need the buoyancy of the water to support the body. It eases the strain on the body so that if there is any specific weakness, it tends to be strengthened slowly when you first start out. Generally speaking, swimmers should ensure that their physical rhythm is in its positive phase when they either train or actually take part in a competition. Good emotional levels would be helpful for a more positive frame of mind at such times.

Short distance running is where competitiveness is of paramount importance at all times. Long distance running suggests the need for the stamina to withstand the calls on the body's reserves and then when and where to strike so that others will be (hopefully) left gasping.

While football needs stamina and a good eye, which suggests the need for intellectual expertise (within the parameters of the game, of course) because it is a team game. While there will always be 'stars' in teams, they must appreciate that they have to be a proper part of their side at all times. Therefore, they have to play together and not for themselves. The object of the game is to win, of course, but not at any price.

Team members should train regularly and as often as possible but these times should always be eased somewhat when the cycles of some of the individuals are in their negative stages or their low periods. Many football managers are aware of the biorhythm system and, while they may not always admit to it (if at all), quite a few will note when their players abilities are at their best.

When a player's rhythms are in the positive phase, they may take on some extra training if there is a need to do so.

Further, if the coach or trainer is able to read and understand what these cycles are all about, then he or she should also be in a position to obtain the charts of the opposing team as well. This will give them plenty of opportunity to study and produce the right strategy to win.

Rugby on the other hand is much more of a specialist game. The team member must know how to compete properly for the ball at a break or a tackle down and burst through tackles.

He or she (please remember that the ladies also play this game most efficiently) also has to keep a scrum drive going for a fellow team member to capitalise on as and when. They have to be extremely quick both in defence or attack and their fitness needs to keep them going to dodge and play all out for two periods of 40 minutes each.

To become fit properly for rugby, players need to be recruited while still fairly young and then trained in such a way as to allow them as much fun as they can deal with along with also learning how to play the game. Rugby demands a special fitness and outlook at all times. The older player must always know how to develop properly for the game.

All sporting activities need each of the three rhythms to be in their positive stages but, obviously, this is not always practicable or possible. A positive physical rhythm with a high or low emotional or intellectual cycle will need careful monitoring. Once again, you should have your personal biorhythm chart set up well in advance because proper planning is essential if you are to succeed in your particular choice of sport.

If all three cycles are in the plus phase, the subject is more than likely to overplay his or her hand. If too much exuberance or over-use of the available energy is exploited, it can lead to an uncontrolled situation. That all three energies are in the right stage is fine, but to control them effectively is yet another task. When all three biorhythms are in their negative stages then only the best efforts are going to mean anything.

While they may not exactly set the world on fire, people can still give of their best and still win with careful planning. With only one or two rhythms in the critical stage, performance will be either brilliant or erratic. Experience suggests that both seem to occur in far too many cases.

Skaters, for example, need to measure their abilities with greater care than most because if they do make a mistake, the environment in which they perform can be quite unforgiving. To fall on ice when stationary is one thing but to do so at speed can cause much more damage with a stronger chance of breaking a leg or an arm.

Recuperation will be over a long period and that, along with all the other considerations to worry about, might well put the skater out of action for a long time, in some cases, for far too long. Ideally, the skater's biorhythms should be in the physically positive phase, together with a good emotional cycle stage for support. While it would help to have the intellectual rhythm in its positive stage as well, this sport has more of a physical and emotional desire to win that drives these people on.

Curiously, many skaters often do their best on a day when their physical cycle is in its critical stage. It seems that it is often a question of that little extra drive that spurs these people on and many have found that this happens on a win or lose day, come what may.

Tennis players know how to balance their biorhythms and they will use a low physical cycle to be cleverly utilised with a positive stage intellectual cycle to cut out distraction. Basically, tennis players have to rely on themselves and their own skills to survive. They can work wonders if they have their personal biorhythm calendars to refer to.

Here in the UK, cricket as a team sport brings each individual under some rather intense pressure at times. While the batsman, bowler, wicket-keeper and fieldsmen can and do all carry out their various responsibilities as individuals, they still have to play more or less independently. Nevertheless, they must also remember that, first and foremost, they are part of a team. Of course, the batting pair have to think as one for running between wickets has to be a practical matter and it is always possible that they may have to share a partnership for quite a long time.

Polo appeals to many people but it is an expensive interest to say the least. It isn't widely known or appreciated that left-handed people need not bother for only right-handed folk may play at any time. The left-handed fraternity were officially banned around the 1930s, mainly for safety reasons.

Shortly after World War II, the rule was relaxed because of a lack of competent players. However, it was proved to be quite a dangerous affair and in 1974 the rule was re-instated by USPA, the ruling body of Polo. To date, there are no left handed players in the official sense but there are a few left hand only teams scattered about here and there.

Water Polo on the other hand demands top rate physical fitness at all times. In a one hour match, a player may be called on to cover as much as four kilometres in distance and must know how to tread water for some time. Players should have a very high level of aerobic style abilities. People should only pursue this when their physical cycle is in the positive phase. The intellectual cycle should also be positive while the emotional rarely seems to count for much in this sport.

Squash has been nominated as the healthiest sport of them all but it is also the cause of many a heart attack as well. This is one hell-for-leather activity that requires a player to be in tip-top condition at all times.

It can cause knee or ankle problems along with the strain that can affect the lower half of the body. Injuries to shoulders are common because the player is surrounded by walls and he or she is liable to bump into a wall or even their fellow competitor when running after the ball to gain points. Thus, people who indulge in this sport should have their physical biorhythm in its positive phase with good support from the other two cycles at all times.

It never pays to ignore these rules; for you can do real damage if you are not 100% fit at the time of a game. It never pays to keep going when you know you should rest and that goes for any sporting activity.

A baseball trainer or coach might find a player who does quite well but only at an average pace for the most of the time. Another search could turn up someone who showed a very high level of ability all the time they were playing. At such times, the biorhythm exponent must try to find people to match these quite different characters. A quite high standard of compatibility will be needed between not only the fellow players but also between the trainers and coaches. This will then enable a far better level of understanding between them all.

There should only be one result of such a study – the winning one – and, remember it doesn't stop at baseball either. Just look at all the different sports we have just covered and how we have discovered which particular rhythm should be in what phase to try to ensure success.

CHAPTER 14

CELEBRITY LIST

This list has been very carefully compiled from the famous, the infamous, the not so well known, the criminal fraternity and those who managed to hit the headlines for a variety of other reasons.

The reader may wish to pursue his or her study of biorhythms by looking up important dates in the lives of some of the people listed below who made or took decisions or who acted in the way that they did.

Claudio Abbado	26 June 1933
Andre Agassi	29 April 1970
Louisa M Alcott	29 November 1832
Princess Alexandra	25 December 1936
Mohammed Ali 1	8 January 1942
Woody Allen	1 December 1935
Ursula Andress	19 March 1938
Prince Andrew	19 February 1960
Julie Andrews	1 October 1935
Jennifer Aniston	11 February 1969
Princess Anne	15 August 1950
Antony Armstrong-Jones	07 March 1930
Paddy Ashdown	27 February 1941
Fred Astaire	10 May 1899
Rowan Atkinson	12 January 1955
Lauren Bacall	16 September 1924

Douglas Bader	21 February 1910
Brigitte Bardot 2	8 September 1934
Ronnie Barker	25 September 1929
David Beckham	2 May 1975
Victoria Beckham	17 April 1974
Sir Thomas Beecham	29 April 1879
Alexander Graham Bell	3 March 1847
Tony Bennett	3 August 1926
Ingrid Bergman	29 August 1917
Justin Bieber	1 March 1994
Tony Blair	6 May 1953
Usain Bolt	21 August 1986
Betty Boothroyd	8 October 1929
Victor Borge	3 January 1909
Ian Botham	24 November 1955
David Bowie	8 January 1947
Julian Bream	15 July 1933
Charles Bronson	3 November 1922
Pierce Brosnan	16 May 1953
Richard Burton	10 November 1925
James Caan	26 March 1939
Marti Caine	26 January 1945
Michael Caine	14 March 1933
Duchess of Cambridge	09 January 1982
David Cameron	9 October 1966
Al Capone	17 January 1899
Pablo Casals	29 December 1876
Roger Casement	1 November 1864
Barbara Castle	6 October 1911
Fidel Castro	13 August 1926
Charles Chaplin	16 April 1889
Prince Charles	14 November 1948
Richard Trenton Chase	23 May 1950
Lorraine Chase	16 July 1951

CELEBRITY LIST

Andrei Chikatilo	16 October 1936
John Cleese	27 October 1939
Bill Clinton	19 August 1946
Hilary Clinton	26 October 1947
Joan Collins	23 May 1933
Sean Connery	25 August 1930
Robin Cook	28 February 1946
Henry Cooper	3 May 1934
Ronnie Corbett	4 December 1930
Simon Cowell	7 October 1959
Marie Curie	7 November 1867
Timothy Dalton	21 March 1946
Jim Davidson	13 December 1953
Bette Davis	5 April 1908
Sammy Davis Jnr	8 December 1925
Doris Day	3 April 1924
James Dean	8 February 1931
Catherine Deneuve	22 October 1943
Johnny Depp	9 June 1963
Diana Princess of Wales	1 July 1961
Charles Dickens	7 February 1812
Walt Disney	5 December 1901
Amanda Donohoe	29 June 1962
Kirk Douglas	9 December 1916
Sir Arthur Conan Doyle	22 May 1859
Fay Dunaway	14 January 1941
Bob Dylan	24 May 1941
Clint Eastwood	31 May 1931
Mary Baker Eddy	16 July 1821
Noel Edmonds	22 December 1948
King Edward VII	9 November 1841
Prince Edward	10 March 1964
Samantha Eggar	3 May 1939
Albert Einstein	14 March 1879

Dwight D Eisenhower	14 October 1890
Queen Elizabeth II	21 April 1926
Queen Elizabeth the Queen Mother	4 August 1900
Ben Elton	3 May 1959
David Essex	23 July 1948
Chris Evans	1 April 1966
Kenny Everett	25 December 1944
Peter Falk	16 September 1927
Albert Fish	19 May 1870
Michael Flatley	16 July 1958
Henry Fonda	16 May 1905
Jane Fonda	21 December 1937
Dame Margo Fonteyn	18 May 1919
Glen Ford	1 May 1916
Bruce Forsyth	22 February 1928
General Franco	4 December 1892
Aretha Franklin	25 March 1942
Lady Antonia Fraser	27 August 1932
Dawn French	11 October 1957
Sir Clement Freud	24 April 1924
Sigmund Freud	6 May 1856
Sir David Frost	7 April 1939
Stephen Fry	24 August 1957
John Wayne Gacy	17 May 1942
Yuri Gagarin	9 March 1934
Greta Garbo	18 September 1905
Judy Garland	10 June 1922
James Garner	7 April 1928
Lesley Garret	10 April 1955
Paul Gascoigne	27 May 1967
Bill Gates	28 October 1955
Bob Geldorf	5 October 1954
King George V	3 June 1865
King George VI	14 December 1895

CELEBRITY LIST

Prince George	22 July 2013
John Glenn	18 July 1921
Gary Glitter	8 May 1934
Hermann Goering	12 January 1893
Michael Grade	8 March 1943
Billy Graham	7 November 1918
Cary Grant	18 January 1904
Hugh Grant	9 September 1960
Larry Grayson	31 August 1923
Germaine Greer	29 January 1939
Sir Alec Guinness	2 April 1914
Gene Hackman	30 January 1931
William Hague	26 March 1961
Tony Hancock	3 May 1924
George Harrison	25 February 1943
Prince Harry	15 September 1984
Goldie Hawn	21 November 1945
Sir Edward Heath	9 July 1916
Audrey Hepburn	4 May 1929
Michael Heseltine	21 March 1933
Wild Bill Hickock	27 May 1837
Damon Hill	17 September 1960
Sir Edmund Hillary	20 July 1919
Alfred Hitchcock	13 August 1899
Adolf Hitler	20 April 1889
Dustin Hoffman	8 August 1937
Harry Houdini	6 April 1874
Jaques Ibert	15 August 1890
Henrik Ibsen	20 March 1828
Vincent d'Indy	27 March 1851
Jeremy Irons	19 September 1948
Eddie Izzard	7 February 1962
Mick Jagger	26 July 1943
Glenda Jackson	9 May 1936

Michael Jackson	29 August 1958
Jesse James	5 September 1882
David Janssen	27 March 1930
David Jason	2 February 1940
Sir Elton John	25 March 1947
Tom Jones	7 June 1940
Janis Joplin	19 January 1943
Carl Jung	26 July 1875
Danny Kaye	18 January 1913
Buster Keaton	4 October 1895
Helen Keller	27 June 1880
Gene Kelly	23 August 1912
Grace Kelly	12 November 1929
Felicity Kendal	25 September 1946
Nigel Kennedy	28 December 1956
Deborah Kerr	30 September 1921
Ben Kingsley	31 December 1943
Henry Kissinger	27 May 1923
Reg Kray (Crime Twins)	24 October 1933
Ronnie Kray (Crime Twins)	24 October 1933
Burt Lancaster	2 November 1913
Angela Lansbury	16 October 1925
Mario Lanza	31 January 1921
Heath Ledger	4 April 1979
Christopher Lee	27 May 1922
John Lennon	9 October 1942
Jerry Lee Lewis	29 September 1935
Liberace	16 May 1919
Abraham Lincoln	12 February 1809
Charles Lindberg	4 February 1902
Maureen Lipman	10 May 1946
Franz Liszt	22 October 1811
Sophia Loren	20 September 1934
Joanna Lumley	1 May 1946

CELEBRITY LIST

Shirley Maclaine	24 April 1934
Paul McCartney	18 June 1942
Madonna (Ciccone)	16 August 1958
John Major	29 March 1943
Nelson Mandela	18 July 1918
Peter Mandelson	21 October 1953
Princess Margaret	21 August 1930
Pippa Middleton	6 September 1983
Edward Miliband	24 December 1969
Spike Milligan	16 April 1918
Bob Monkhouse	1 June 1928
Patrick Moore	4 March 1923
Roger Moore	14 October 1927
Eric Morecambe	14 May 1926
Kate Moss	16 January 1974
Lord Louis Mountbatten	25 June 1900
Audie Murphy	20 June 1924
Andy Murray	15 May 1987
Pete Murray	19 September 1925
Admiral Lord Nelson	29 September 1758
Anthony Newley	24 September 1931
Paul Newman	26 January 1925
Jack Nicklaus	21 January 1940
Vaslaw Nijinsky	28 February 1890
Leonard Nimoy	26 March 1931
Richard Nixon	9 January 1913
Rudolph Nureyev	17 March 1938
Barack Obama	4 August 1961
Merle Oberon	19 February 1911
Des O'Connor	12 January 1932
Paul O'Grady	14 June 1955
Maureen O'Hara	17 August 1921
Gary Oldman	21 March 1958
Lord Olivier	22 May 1907

Jacqueline Onassis	28 July 1929
Ryan O'Neal	20 April 1949
George Orwell	25 June 1903
Richard O'Sullivan	7 May 1944
Peter O'Toole	2 August 1933
Al Pacino	25 April 1940
Camilla Parker-Bowles	17 July 1947
Dolly Parton	19 January 1946
Prince Philip	10 June 1921
Leslie Phillips	20 April 1924
Brad Pitt	18 December 1963
Edgar Allen Poe	19 January 1809
Sidney Poitier	20 February 1927
Roman Polanski	18 August 1933
Enoch Powell	16 June 1912
John Prescott	31 May 1938
Elvis Presley	8 January 1935
Andre Previn	6 April 1929
Vincent Price	27 May 1911
Vladimir Putin	7 October 1952
Mary Quant	11 February 1934
Caroline Quentin	11 July 1959
Sir Anthony Quayle	7 September 1913
Anthony Quinn	21 April 1916
Roger Quilter	1 November 1877
Dennis Rader	9 March 1945
Ronald Reagan	6 February 1911
Robert Redford	18 August 1937
Vanessa Redgrave	30 January 1937
Sir Cliff Richard	14 October 1940
Dame Diana Rigg	20 July 1938
Anita Roddick	23 October 1942
Ginger Rogers	16 July 1911
Mickey Rooney	23 September 1920

CELEBRITY LIST

Diana Ross 2	6 March 1944
JK Rowling (Joanne Kathleen)	31 July 1965
Telly Savalas	21 January 1924
Jennifer Saunders	12 July 1958
Peter Sellers	8 September 1925
Frank Sinatra	12 December 1915
William Shatner	22 March 1931
Dr Harold Shipman	14 January 1946
Delia Smith	18 June 1951
Mel Smith	3 December 1952
Will Smith	25 September 1968
Boris Spassky	30 January 1937
Stephen Spielberg	18 December 1946
Barbara Stanwyck	16 July 1907
Ringo Starr	7 July 1940
Tommy Steele	17 December 1936
Barbra Streisand	24 April 1942
Peter Stringfellow	17 October 1940
ALAN (Lord) Sugar	24 March 1947
Gloria Swanson	27 March 1899
Eric Sykes	4 May 1923
Chris Tarrant	10 October 1946
Margaret Thatcher	13 October 1925
Dame Kiri Te Kanawa	6 March 1946
Terry Thomas	14 July 1911
Jeremy Thorpe	29 April 1929
Marshall Tito	25 May 1892
Mel Torme	13 September 1925
Paul Tortelier	21 March 1914
Lana Turner	8 February 1920
Twiggy	19 September 1949
Leslie Uggams	25 May 1943
Ulanova	10 January 1910
Liv Ullman	16 December 1939

Tracy Ullman	30 December 1959
Captain Charles Upham	21 September 1908
Stanley Unwin	7 June 1911
Mary Ure	18 February 1933
Peter Ustinov	16 April 1921
Rudolph Valentino	6 May 1895
Eamon de Valera	14 October 1882
Frankie Vaughan	3 February 1928
Robert Vaughan	22 November 1932
Ralph Vaughan Williams	12 October 1872
Jules Verne	8 February 1828
Queen Victoria	24 May 1819
Gore Vidal	3 October 1925
Lindsay Wagner	22 June 1949
Clint Walker	30 May 1927
Sir Barnes Wallis	26 September 1887
John Wayne	26 May 1907
Ruby Wax	19 April 1953
Raquel Welch	5 September 1942
Orson Welles	6 May 1915
Fred West	29 September 1941
Rose (Rosemary) West	29 November 1946
Oscar Wilde	16 October 1854
Prince William	21 June 1982
Kenneth Williams	22 February 1926
Barbara Windsor	6 August 1937
Duke of Windsor	23 June 1894
Duchess of Windsor	19 June 1896
Oprah Winfrey	29 January 1954
Ernie Wise	27 November 1925
Victoria Wood	19 May 1953
Anthony Worral-Thompson	1 May 1952
Aileen Wuornos	29 February 1956
Paula Yates	24 April 1960

Michael York	27 March 1942
Susannah York	9 January 1942
Andrew Young	12 March 1922
Gig Young	4 November 1917
Jimmy Young	21 September 1921
Darryl F Zanuck	5 September 1905
Franco Zefferelli	12 February 1923
Ferdinand Zeppelin	8 July 1838
Catherine Zeta-Jones	25 September 1969
Mai Zetterling	24 May 1925
Efrem Zimbalist Jnr	30 November 1923
Emile Zola	2 April 1840
Pinchas Zuckerman	16 July 1948

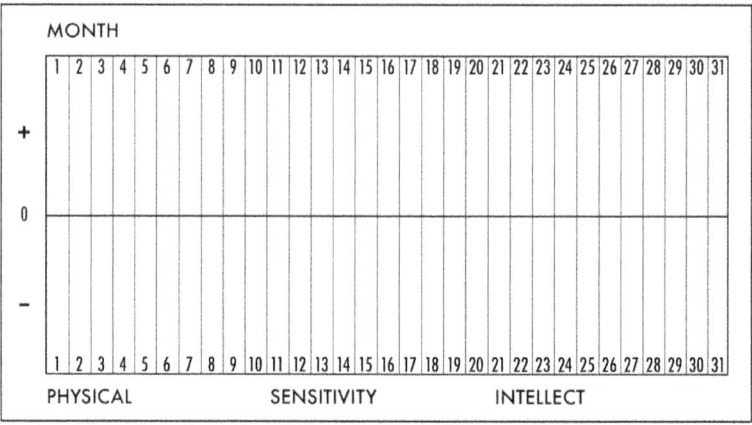
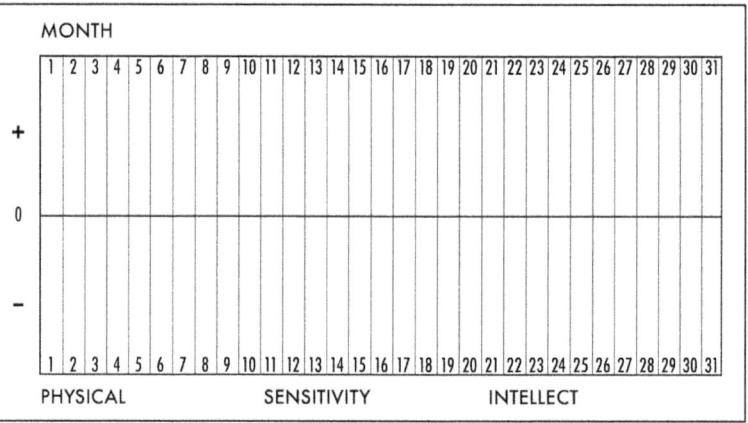
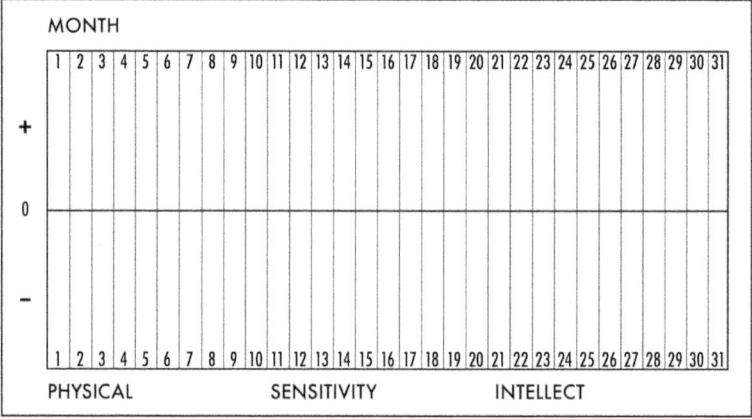

Lightning Source UK Ltd.
Milton Keynes UK
UKHW021454110521
383373UK00004B/42